RICHARD H. HAUG, DDS, CONSULTING EDITOR

ATLAS OF THE ORAL AND MAXILLOFACIAL SURGERY CLINICS
OF NORTH AMERICA

Peripheral Trigeminal Nerve Injury, Repair, and Regeneration

Martin B. Steed, DDS, GUEST EDITOR

W.B. SAUNDERS COMPANY
A Division of Elsevier Inc.
PHILADELPHIA LONDON TORONTO MONTREAL SYDNEY TOKYO

W.B. SAUNDERS COMPANY
A Division of Elsevier Inc.

1600 John F. Kennedy Boulevard, Suite 1800 ⟩ Philadelphia, Pennsylvania 19103-2899
http://www.oralmaxsurgeryatlas.theclinics.com

ATLAS OF THE ORAL AND MAXILLOFACIAL SURGERY CLINICS OF NORTH AMERICA March 2011 Editor: John Vassallo; j.vassallo@elsevier.com Development Editor: Donald Mumford	Volume 19, Number 1 ISSN 1061-3315 ISBN-13: 978-1-4557-0421-7

© **2011 Elsevier Inc. All rights reserved.**

This journal and the individual contributions contained in it are protected under copyright by Elsevier, and the following terms and conditions apply to their use:

Photocopying
Single photocopies of single articles may be made for personal use as allowed by national copyright laws. Permission of the Publisher and payment of a fee is required for all other photocopying, including multiple or systematic copying, copying for advertising or promotional purposes, resale, and all forms of document delivery. Special rates are available for educational institutions that wish to make photocopies for non-profit educational classroom use. For information on how to seek permission visit www.elsevier.com/permissions or call: (+44) 1865 843830 (UK)/(+1) 215 239 3804 (USA).

Derivative Works
Subscribers may reproduce tables of contents or prepare lists of articles including abstracts for internal circulation within their institutions. Permission of the Publisher is required for resale or distribution outside the institution. Permission of the Publisher is required for all other derivative works, including compilations and translations (please consult www.elsevier.com/permissions).

Electronic Storage or Usage
Permission of the Publisher is required to store or use electronically any material contained in this journal, including any article or part of an article (please consult www.elsevier.com/permissions). Except as outlined above, no part of this publication may be reproduced, stored in a retrieval system or transmitted in any form or by any means, electronic, mechanical, photocopying, recording or otherwise, without prior written permission of the Publisher.

Notice
No responsibility is assumed by the Publisher for any injury and/or damage to persons or property as a matter of products liability, negligence or otherwise, or from any use or operation of any methods, products, instructions or ideas contained in the material herein. Because of rapid advances in the medical sciences, in particular, independent verification of diagnoses and drug dosages should be made. Although all advertising material is expected to conform to ethical (medical) standards, inclusion in this publication does not constitute a guarantee or endorsement of the quality or value of such product or of the claims made of it by its manufacturer.

Reprints. For copies of 100 or more of articles in this publication, please contact the Commercial Reprints Department, Elsevier Inc., 360 Park Avenue South, New York, NY 10010-1710. Tel.: 212-633-3812; Fax: 212-462-1935; E-mail: reprints@elsevier.com.

Atlas of the Oral and Maxillofacial Surgery Clinics of North America (ISSN 1061-3315) is published biannually by Elsevier, 360 Park Avenue South, New York, NY 10010-1710. Months of issue are March and September. Periodicals postage paid at New York, NY and additional mailing offices. Subscription prices are $383.00 for international individual, $312.00 for US individual; $188.00 for international student, $153.00 for US student; $364.00 for international institution, $322.00 for US institution. Foreign air speed delivery is included in all *Clinics* subscription prices. All prices are subject to change without notice. POSTMASTER: Send address changes to *Atlas of the Oral and Maxillofacial Surgery Clinics of North America*, Health Sciences Division, Subscription Customer Service, 3251 Riverport Lane, Maryland Heights, MO 63043. Tel: 1-800-654-2452 (U.S. and Canada); 314-447-8871 (outside U.S. and Canada). Fax: 314-417-8029. E-mail: journalscustomerservice-usa@elsevier.com (for print support); journalsonlinesupport-usa@elsevier.com (for online support).

Atlas of the Oral and Maxillofacial Surgery Clinics of North America is covered in *MEDLINE/PubMed (Index Medicus)*.

Printed in the United States of America.

PERIPHERAL TRIGEMINAL NERVE INJURY, REPAIR, AND REGENERATION

CONSULTING EDITOR

RICHARD H. HAUG, DDS, Carolinas Center for Oral Health, Charlotte, North Carolina

GUEST EDITOR

MARTIN B. STEED, DDS, Assistant Professor and Residency Program Director, Division of Oral and Maxillofacial Surgery, Department of Surgery, Emory University School of Medicine, Atlanta, Georgia

CONTRIBUTORS

SHAHROKH C. BAGHERI, DMD, MD, FACS, Private Practice, Georgia Oral and Facial Surgery, Marietta; Chief, Division of Oral and Maxillofacial Surgery, Department of Surgery, Northside Hospital; Assistant Clinical Professor, Department of Surgery, School of Medicine, Emory University, Atlanta; Clinical Associate Professor, Department of Oral and Maxillofacial Surgery, School of Dentistry, Medical College of Georgia, Augusta, Georgia

RAVI V. BELLAMKONDA, PhD, GCC Distinguished Scholar and Professor of Biomedical Engineering, Neurological Biomaterials and Therapeutics, Wallace H. Coulter Department of Biomedical Engineering, Georgia Institute of Technology/Emory University, Atlanta, Georgia

GEORGE BLAKEY III, DMD, Associate Professor, Department of Oral and Maxillofacial Surgery, University of North Carolina, Chapel Hill, North Carolina

GREG K. ESSICK, DDS, PhD, Professor, Department of Prosthodontics, University of North Carolina, Chapel Hill, North Carolina

ANTONIA KOLOKYTHAS, DDS, Assistant Professor and Director of Research, Department of Oral and Maxillofacial Surgery, University of Illinois at Chicago, Chicago, Illinois

ROGER A. MEYER, DDS, MS, MD, FACS, Director, Maxillofacial Consultations Ltd, Greensboro, Georgia

MICHAEL MILORO, DMD, MD, FACS, Professor, Department Head, and Program Director, Department of Oral and Maxillofacial Surgery, University of Illinois at Chicago, Chicago, Illinois

VIVEK MUKHATYAR, BS, Graduate Student, Wallace H. Coulter Department of Biomedical Engineering, Georgia Institute of Technology/Emory University, Atlanta, Georgia

CEIB PHILLIPS, MPH, PhD, Professor, Department of Orthodontics, University of North Carolina, Chapel Hill, North Carolina

DANIEL B. RODRIGUES, DDS, Former Fellow in Oral and Maxillofacial Surgery, Department of Oral and Maxillofacial Surgery, Baylor University Medical Center, Texas A&M University Health Science Center, Baylor College of Dentistry, Dallas, Texas; Private Practice, Salvador, Brazil

MARTIN B. STEED, DDS, Assistant Professor and Residency Program Director, Division of Oral and Maxillofacial Surgery, Department of Surgery, Emory University School of Medicine, Atlanta, Georgia

CHANDRA VALMIKINATHAN, PhD, Postdoctoral Fellow, Wallace H. Coulter Department of Biomedical Engineering, Georgia Institute of Technology/Emory University, Atlanta, Georgia

LARRY M. WOLFORD, DMD, Clinical Professor, Department of Oral and Maxillofacial Surgery, Texas A&M University Health Science Center, Baylor College of Dentistry; Private Practice, Baylor University Medical Center, Dallas, Texas

VINCENT B. ZICCARDI, DDS, MD, Professor and Chair, Department of Oral and Maxillofacial Surgery, New Jersey Dental School, University of Medicine and Dentistry of New Jersey, Newark, New Jersey

PERIPHERAL TRIGEMINAL NERVE INJURY, REPAIR, AND REGENERATION

CONTENTS

Preface: Peripheral Trigeminal Nerve Injury, Repair, and Regeneration   vii
Martin B. Steed

Peripheral Nerve Response to Injury   1
Martin B. Steed

Clinical Evaluation of Peripheral Trigeminal Nerve Injuries   15
Roger A. Meyer and Shahrokh C. Bagheri

Inferior Alveolar and Lingual Nerve Imaging   35
Michael Miloro and Antonia Kolokythas

Management of Mandibular Nerve Injuries from Dental Implants   47
Shahrokh C. Bagheri and Roger A. Meyer

Nerve Injuries from Mandibular Third Molar Removal   63
Roger A. Meyer and Shahrokh C. Bagheri

Microsurgical Techniques for Repair of the Inferior Alveolar and Lingual Nerves   79
Vincent B. Ziccardi

Autogenous Grafts/Allografts/Conduits for Bridging Peripheral Trigeminal Nerve Gaps   91
Larry M. Wolford and Daniel B. Rodrigues

Sensory Retraining: A Cognitive Behavioral Therapy for Altered Sensation   109
Ceib Phillips, George Blakey III, and Greg K. Essick

Advances in Bioengineered Conduits for Peripheral Nerve Regeneration   119
Martin B. Steed, Vivek Mukhatyar, Chandra Valmikinathan, and
Ravi V. Bellamkonda

FORTHCOMING ISSUES

September 2011

Current Concepts in TMJ Surgery
Gregory M. Ness, DDS, *Guest Editor*

March 2012

Virtual Technologies in Oral and Maxillofacial Surgery
Gary P. Orentlicher, DMD, *Guest Editor*

PREVIOUS ISSUES

September 2010

Combined Craniomaxillofacial and Neurosurgical Procedures
Ramon L. Ruiz, DMD, MD, and
Jogi V. Pattisapu, MD, *Guest Editors*

March 2010

Management of the Airway
Henry H. Rowshan, DDS, MAJ, USA, and
Dale A. Baur, DDS, MD, *Guest Editors*

September 2009

Cleft Surgery: Repair of the Lip, Palate, and Alveolus
G.E. Ghali, DDS, MD, FACS, *Guest Editor*

RELATED INTEREST
Neurosurgery Clinics of North America,
January 2009 (Vol. 20, No. 1)
Peripheral Nerves: Injuries
Robert J. Spinner, MD, and Christopher J. Winfree, MD,
Guest Editors

The Clinics are now available online!

Access your subscription at
www.theclinics.com

Preface
Peripheral Trigeminal Nerve Injury, Repair, and Regeneration

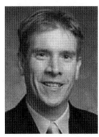

Martin B. Steed, DDS
Guest Editor

The illustrative nature of this *Atlas of the Oral and Maxillofacial Surgery Clinics of North America* lends itself extremely well to the discussion of injury to the peripheral branches of the trigeminal nerve. Injuries to the lingual nerve and inferior alveolar nerve are by their very nature difficult to visualize and this contributes to our diagnostic and therapeutic dilemmas. This issue's focus is primarily on the specific branches of the mandibular or third division of the trigeminal nerve. With the diagrams, photos, and figures provided by this edition's authors, it is my hope that maxillofacial surgeons will be provided with a clearer and more precise look at the nerves that they work so closely with, and around, each day. The more sophisticated our knowledge is of nerve injury, peripheral nerve repair, and peripheral nerve regeneration, the better our ability will be to provide future patients with optimal care.

Dr Goran Lundborg wrote in 1988 that "Still, our approach to peripheral nerve lesions tends to be remarkably non-biological. The surgical procedure for treatment of nerve severance remains basically a matter of preparing the nerve ends adequately, placing sutures in the right positions and using the right optical magnification. The development of microsurgical techniques has helped to improve considerably the results in selected situations. However, we lack a corresponding development of techniques for controlling and manipulating the local microenvironment when surgical techniques cannot be further refined." Almost a quarter of a century later, the same need remains.

These future advances in restoring patients with peripheral nerve injuries to improved outcomes will take place on the "biological battleground" which rages beyond the magnified view of the microscope. Optimizing the body's own ability to regenerate peripheral nerves through therapeutic manipulation of the response to injury at the cellular level has the potential to keep more neurons viable, encourage their axons to cross longer gaps, and provide more precise directional regeneration.

In few fields is the need for translational research more crucial to enable us to provide better care for our patients. Bridging the gap between basic scientists and clinicians is without doubt the answer to bridging the gap at nerve transections. It is my hope that this atlas will stimulate future oral and maxillofacial surgeons to contribute to that end.

Martin B. Steed, DDS
Division of Oral and Maxillofacial Surgery
Department of Surgery
Emory University School of Medicine
1365 Clifton Road, Suite 2300 B
Atlanta, GA 30322, USA

E-mail address: msteed@emory.edu

Peripheral Nerve Response to Injury

Martin B. Steed, DDS

Division of Oral and Maxillofacial Surgery, Department of Surgery, Emory University School of Medicine, 1365 Clifton Road, Suite 2300 B, Atlanta, GA 30322, USA

Injury to the peripheral trigeminal nerve results in various extents of nerve fiber injury. The consequences to the patient are almost always detrimental and can influence the patient's ability to eat comfortably, taste, manage oral secretions, and speak clearly. Many lingual and inferior alveolar nerve injuries require no surgical intervention and the patient's sensation returns to normal with time. Other injuries show incomplete or no improvement with time. To compare these 2 types of clinical scenarios, the surgeon must first understand the response of the peripheral nerve to injury. The fate of the axons and/or the surrounding architecture of the nerve components is critical for recovery after injury. The healing of nerve injuries is unique within the body because it is a process of cellular repair rather than cell division or mitosis. The nerve cells at the site do not increase in number after an injury, but attempt to restore the axoplasmic volume and continuity of the original neurons.

Anatomy

A sophisticated understanding of the anatomy of the peripheral nerve is beneficial to comprehending the series of events that takes place after an injury. A normal polyfascicular trigeminal nerve is shown in Fig. 1. The components of the peripheral nerve include connective tissue, blood vessels, and the basic unit of the peripheral nerve: an axon and its associated Schwann cells. The nerve trunk represents a composite tissue constructed for the purpose of maintaining continuity, nutrition, and protection of these basic units, which require a continuous energy supply to allow for impulse conductivity and axonal transport.

Connective Tissue

The connective tissue subdivisions provide the framework around and within the nerve. The resulting architecture consists of an external and internal epineurium, and a perineurium surrounding each fascicle, in which are contained multiple axons surrounded by endoneurium. A fourth subdivision includes a mesoneurium that consists of loose areolar tissue continuous with the epineurium and the surrounding tissue bed. The mesoneurium allows the nerve to move a certain distance longitudinally within the surrounding tissue.

The outer connective tissue layer of the nerve is the external epineurium, which is a supporting and protective connective tissue made up primarily of collagen and elastic fibers (Fig. 2). The internal epineurium is the structure that invests the fascicles, which contain the nerve fibers. Usually, several fascicles are grouped together in bundles, constituting well-defined subunits of the nerve trunk. Fascicles vary in size and quantity depending primarily on whether the region in question is at the proximal or distal site of the nerve. Both the lingual and inferior alveolar nerves are polyfascicular. The lingual nerve contains 15 to 18 fascicles at the region adjacent the mandibular third molar, whereas the inferior alveolar nerve contains 18 to 21 fascicles within the angle of the mandible.

The author has nothing to disclose.
E-mail address: msteed@emory.edu

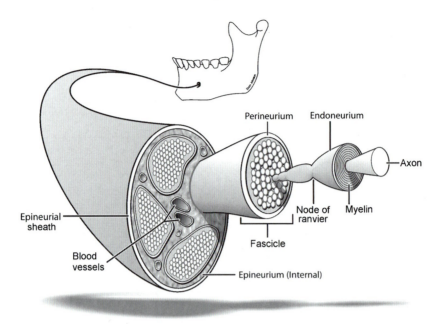

Fig. 1. Cross-sectional view of the peripheral trigeminal nerve internal anatomy. (*Courtesy of* Don Johnson, Emory University, Atlanta, GA.)

Each fascicle is surrounded by perineurium, a lamellated sheath with considerable tensile mechanical strength and elasticity (Fig. 3). The perineurium is made up of collagen fibers dispersed among perineural cells and acts as a diffusion barrier as a result of its selective permeability, separating the endoneurial space within it from the surrounding tissues. This separation preserves the ionic environment within the fascicle.

The nerve fibers are closely packed within endoneurial connective tissue (endoneurium) inside each fascicle (Figs. 4 and 5). The endoneurium is composed of a loose gelatinous collagen matrix.

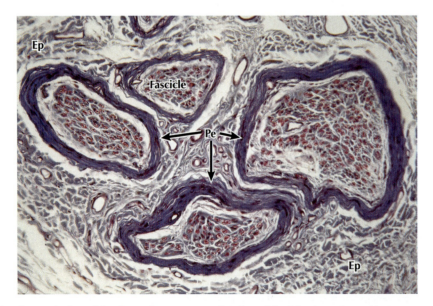

Fig. 2. Light micrograph of a peripheral nerve in transverse section. Several fascicles that make up this nerve are enveloped by the connective tissue of the epineurium (Ep) that merges imperceptibly with the surrounding loose connective tissue, the mesoneurium. A more deeply stained perineurium (Pe) encloses the fascicles. Each fascicle consists of a large number of nerve fibers that are embedded in a more delicate endoneurium (not well defined at this level of magnification). Magnification ×200, Masson trichrome. (*From* Netter illustration from www.netterimages.com. © Elsevier Inc. All rights reserved.)

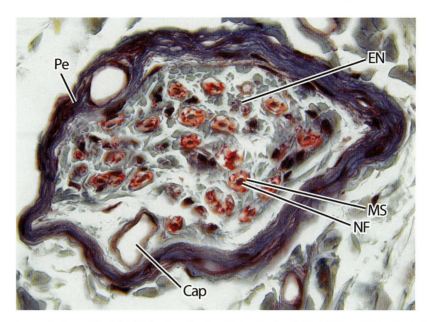

Fig. 3. Light micrograph of a nerve fascicle at higher magnification. The perineurium (Pe) is dark blue and the endoneurium (EN) light blue. Nerve fibers (NF) are densely stained structures surrounded by a myelin sheath (MS), which is red. A capillary (Cap) is shown. Magnification ×465, Masson trichrome. (*From* Netter illustration from www.netterimages.com. © Elsevier Inc. All rights reserved.)

Blood Supply

The axon of each neuron requires a continuous energy supply for impulse transmission and axonal transport. This energy is provided by extrinsic and an intrinsic vascular systems, which are interconnected. The extrinsic vessels enter the mesoneurium and communicate with the epineurial space via the vasa nervorum. A plexus develops at this level and runs longitudinally (Fig. 6). Close

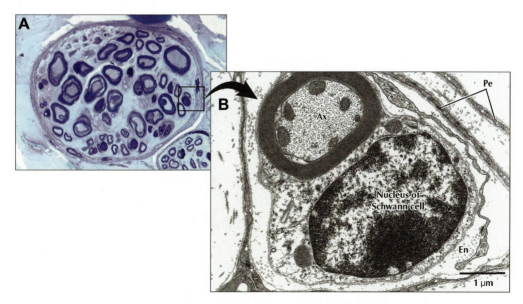

Fig. 4. (*A*) Light micrograph of a peripheral nerve fascicle in transverse section. Osmium fixation shows well-preserved myelin sheaths of nerve fibers. Nerve fibers vary in diameter, and perineurium surrounds the fascicle (Toluidine blue, magnification ×600; semithin plastic section). (*B*) Electron micrograph of a myelinated nerve fiber and its associated Schwann cell in transverse section. The myelinated nerve fibre axoplasm (Ax) contains cytoskeletal elements and mitochondria that parallel its long axis. The Schwann cell, sectioned at the level of its nucleus, is enveloped externally by a basal lamina. Flattened perineurial cells (Pe) and collagen fibrils of the endoneurium (En) are also seen (magnification ×16,800).

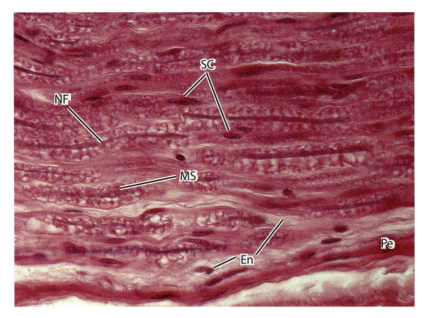

Fig. 5. Light micrograph of peripheral nerve in longitudinal section. Nerve fibers (NF), the slender deeply stained threads, pursue a wavy course. Myelin sheaths (MS) appear vacuolated because of high lipid content and the effects of paraffin embedding on the tissue sample. Schwann cells (SC) have elongated nuclei. They are indistinguishable from the nuclei of fibroblasts of the delicate endoneurium (En) that invests the individual nerve fibers. A deeply stained perineurium (Pe) surrounds the nerve fascicle externally. Magnification ×700, hematoxylin-eosin. (*From* Netter illustration from www.netterimages.com. © Elsevier Inc. All rights reserved.)

examination of the fascicles reveals a large number of epineurial vascular branches, supplying each fascicle in a segmental manner, so that each fascicle is vascularly analogous to a complete axon (Fig. 7 top).

The plexus enters the endoneurium through the perineurium at an oblique angle to anastomose with the intrinsic circulation that surrounds each fascicle. The oblique passage of vessels through the inner perineurial membrane is a site of potential circulatory compromise within the intrafascicular tissue.

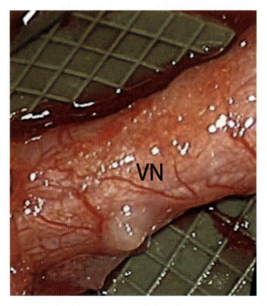

Fig. 6. A lingual nerve under microscopic magnification showing the vasa nervorum (VN). Large longitudinally oriented intrinsic epineurial arteriolar and venular vessels can be seen deep to this plexus.

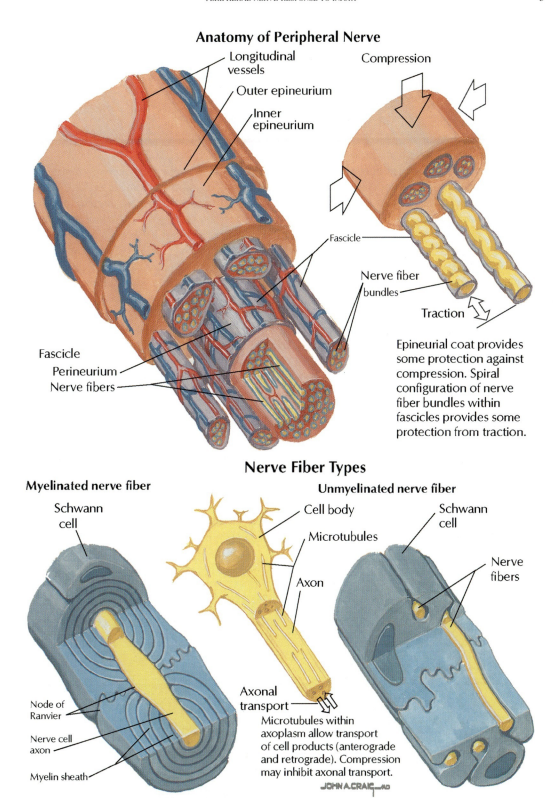

Fig. 7. Anatomy of a peripheral nerve. Both the interconnected (intrinsic) vascular components and the nerve fiber types (myelinated and unmyelinated) are shown. Vessels are abundant in all layers of the nerve, forming a pattern of longitudinally oriented vessels. Vessels penetrate the perineurium following an oblique course. Myelinated and unmyelinated axons are shown (*bottom*). A single Schwann cell can envelop multiple unmyelinated axons and concentrically wrap its cell membrane around an axon to form a myelinated fiber. (*From* Netter illustration from www.netterimages.com. © Elsevier Inc. All rights reserved.)

Nerve Fibers

A neuron consists of a nerve cell body and its processes. There are several dendrites associated with the cell body and 1 long extension: an axon that travels to an end organ with branches terminating in peripheral synaptic terminals.

Nerve fibers can be either myelinated or unmyelinated (see Fig. 7 bottom). Sensory and motor nerves contain both types of fibers in a ratio of 4 unmyelinated to 1 myelinated.

Unmyelinated fibers are made up of several axons enclosed by a single Schwann cell (Fig. 8). Unmyelinated axons are small in diameter, usually averaging 0.15 to 2.0 μm.

The axons of a myelinated fiber are individually wrapped by a single Schwann cell that has laid down a laminar myelin sheath (Fig. 9). The center of a myelinated fiber is made up of cytoplasm (axoplasm) with associated cytoskeletal elements surrounded by a membrane (axolemma). A concentric sheath of myelin and a Schwann cell surround this membrane (Fig. 10). A thin basal lamina invests the interdigitating processes of Schwann cells. At the junction between 2 Schwann cells, the axolemma becomes exposed at a gap called a node of Ranvier (Fig. 11). The propagation of an action potential along the axon jumps from node to node over the insulated areas covered with myelin in the process of saltatory conduction, which provides for more rapid propagation along the axon. As a result, myelinated fibers are able to conduct an impulse at a speed up to 150 m/s, whereas unmyelinated fibers propagate impulses at speeds of 2 to 2.5 m/s.

The cell bodies of the peripheral trigeminal nerve including the lingual and inferior alveolar nerve are contained within the trigeminal ganglion (also called the semilunar ganglion) (Fig. 12). The trigeminal ganglion is analogous to the dorsal root ganglia of the spinal cord, which contain the cell bodies of incoming sensory fibers from the rest of the body. These nerve cells may have axons that extend for a distance corresponding to thousands of cell body diameters, which imposes special requirements on the communication systems between the proximal and distal regions of the cell. To meet these requirements, the neuron has unique systems of anterograde as well as retrograde intracellular transport. These transport mechanisms are involved in the response to injury.

Overview of response to injury

If axonal continuity is maintained after an injury, then functional recovery may be complete, although the time needed may vary. Clinically useful injury grading systems have been developed

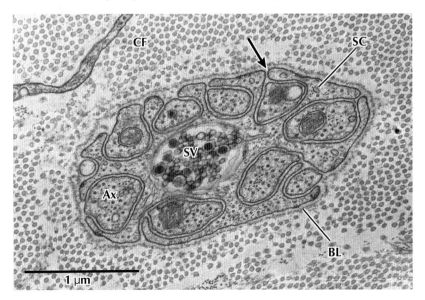

Fig. 8. Electron micrograph of a Schwann cell associated with several unmyelinated nerve fibers in transverse section. Nerve fibers (Ax) occupy channel-like invaginations of Schwann cell cytoplasm (SC). Most nerve fibers contain neurofibrils and microtubules. One nerve fiber in the center contains clear, dense core synaptic vesicles (SV). A basal lamina (BL) covers the outer aspect of the Schwann cell, and a mesaxon is indicated (*arrow*). Surrounding endoneurial connective tissue contains collagen fibrils (CF). 33,000×. (*From* Netter illustration from www.netterimages.com. © Elsevier Inc. All rights reserved.)

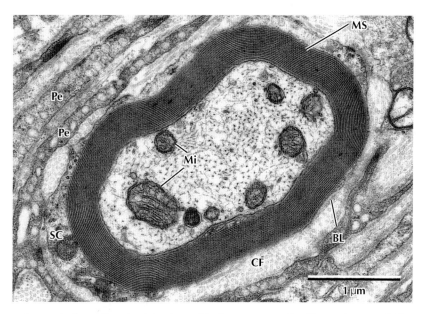

Fig. 9. Electron micrograph of a myelinated peripheral nerve fiber in transverse section. The axon is surrounded by a myelin sheath (MS) composed of multiple lamellae formed by the plasma membrane of a Schwann cell. A thin rim of Schwann cell cytoplasm (SC) envelops the myelin and is invested externally by a thin basal lamina (BL). Collagen fibers (CF) of the endoneurium and flattened perineurial cells (Pe) are in the surrounding area. The nerve axoplasm contains mitochondria (Mi), neurofilaments, and a few microtubules. Magnification ×30,000. (*From* Netter illustration from www.netterimages.com. © Elsevier Inc. All rights reserved.)

that allow correlation of the histologic changes occurring after nerve injury with patient symptoms. The most widely used systems are those developed by Seddon and Sunderland (Fig. 13 bottom). Seddon divided the nerve injuries by severity into 3 broad categories: neurapraxia, axonotmesis, and neurotmesis. For example, a moderate nerve compression injury to the lingual nerve from retraction during a surgical extraction of a third molar can be classified as a neurapraxia (Sunderland type I injury), indicating a local conduction block with good chances for functional recovery within weeks

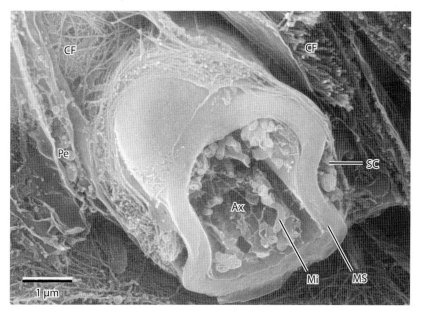

Fig. 10. High-resolution scanning electron micrograph of a myelinated peripheral nerve fiber fractured in the transverse plane. The axon, fractured open, reveals mitochondria (Mi) and cytoskeletal elements in the axoplasm (Ax). A peripheral rim of Schwann cell cytoplasm (SC) is outside the myelin sheath (MS). Collagen fibrils (CF) of the surrounding endoneurium can be seen. A flattened perineurial cell (Pe) is also fractured open. Magnification ×15,000. (*From* Netter illustration from www.netterimages.com. © Elsevier Inc. All rights reserved.)

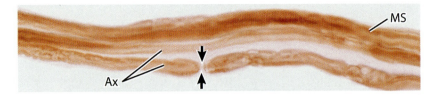

Fig. 11. Light micrograph of teased myelinated nerve fibers showing a node of Ranvier. The axon (Ax) is the central pale region in each fiber. Myelin sheaths (MS), visible when fixed and stained with osmium, appear as dark linear densities. A node of Ranvier (*arrows*) is indicated. Magnification ×500, osmium. (*From* Netter illustration from www.netterimages.com. © Elsevier Inc. All rights reserved.)

or months. Axonotmesis (Sunderland II) occurs when there is complete interruption of the nerve axon and surrounding myelin, whereas the perineurium and epineurium are preserved. For example, if there is a more significant injury, the axonal continuity may eventually be interrupted, resulting in degeneration of the distal axonal segment and complete denervation (see Fig. 13 top). Recovery is possible in such injuries because of the remaining uninjured mesenchymal latticework that provides a path for subsequent sprouting axons to reinnervate their target organ. Neurotmesis (Sunderland V), the complete transection of a nerve trunk, represents a more serious clinical situation. Functional loss is complete and recovery is unlikely.

Peripheral nerve response to transection has been shown to be a complex but finely regulated sequence of events intended to remove the damaged tissue and begin the reparative process. Before regeneration of nerve fibers can begin, a series of degenerative processes must take place. The healing of nerve injuries is unique within the body because it is a process of cellular repair rather than tissue repair; the nerve cells do not undergo mitoses. The number of nerve cells (neurons) does not increase, but the amputated nerve cell regains its original axoplasmic volume by sending out new processes to the end organ target. Although the number of neurons does not increase, the repair of each cell takes place in an environment of intense cellular proliferation. The cells that do show evidence of proliferation include Schwann cells, endothelial cells, and fibroblasts.

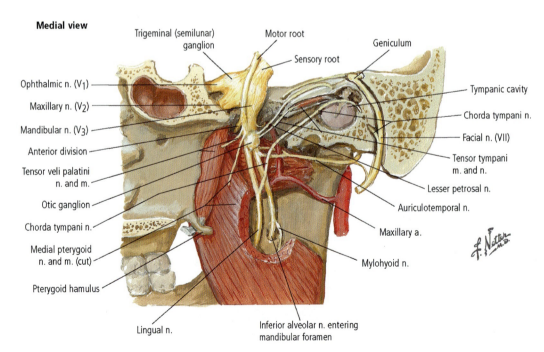

Fig. 12. Medial view of the trigeminal nerve. The cell bodies of the peripheral trigeminal nerve, including the lingual and inferior alveolar nerve, are contained within the trigeminal ganglion (also called the semilunar ganglion). The trigeminal ganglion is analogous to the dorsal root ganglia of the spinal cord, which contain the cell bodies of incoming sensory fibers from the rest of the body. (*From* Netter illustration from www.netterimages.com. © Elsevier Inc. All rights reserved.)

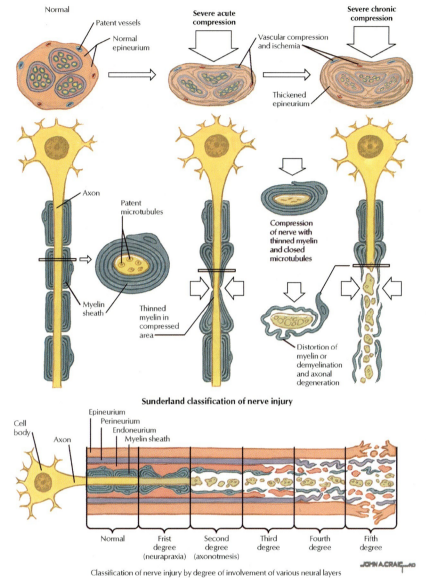

Fig. 13. Nerve injury spectrum from compression and Sunderland classification of nerve injury. A normal peripheral nerve is represented as well as a nerve that has undergone severe acute compression with resultant thinning of the myelin sheath and closure of microtubules. After severe chronic compression, demyelination can result with concurrent axonal degeneration. The Sunderland classification scheme is shown in longitudinal section showing the inside-out histologic progression of injury with a fifth degree injury representing a neurotmesis defined as complete nerve transection. (*From* Netter illustration from www.netterimages.com. © Elsevier Inc. All rights reserved.)

Axonal degeneration

A normal myelinated axon and its components (cell body, myelin, Schwann cells, basal lamina) are depicted in Fig. 14. Within hours after an axonal transection, a series of events takes place at the site of injury, at the distal and proximal portion of the axon, and at the cell body of the neuron.

Changes in the neuronal cell body and in nerve fibers proximal to the site of injury depend both on the severity of the injury and the proximity of the injury to the cell body. The nerve cell body itself reacts to axonal injury in a predictable fashion. Within 6 hours of injury, the nucleus migrates to the periphery of the cell body and Nissl granules (rough endoplasmic reticulum) break up and disperse in a process called chromatolysis. Simultaneously, there is a significant proliferative response of perineurial glial (support) cells, most likely signaled by the process of chromatolysis.

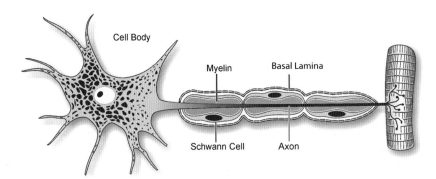

Fig. 14. A normal myelinated axon associated with a longitudinal chain of Schwann cells and enclosed within a continuous basal lamina. (*Courtesy of* Don Johnson, Emory University, Atlanta, GA.)

Distal to the injury, a series of molecular and cellular events (some are simultaneous, whereas others are consecutive) that are collectively termed wallerian degeneration (Fig. 15) are triggered throughout the distal nerve stump and within a small reactive zone at the tip of the proximal stump. In wallerian (or anterograde) degeneration, the primary histologic change involves physical fragmentation of both axons and myelin. Ultrastructurally, both neurotubules and neurofilaments become disarrayed. Within hours of physical interruption, the ends of the axon are sealed. Anterograde axoplasmic transport continues within the proximal stump and retrograde axonal transport continues for several days. As a consequence, the ends of the sealed axons swell as they fill with organelles that are unable to progress beyond the site of the discontinuity. Until recently, it was assumed that axons degenerated because they were no longer supported by their cell bodies. More recent studies have revealed that disconnected axons destroy themselves likely through an early chain of events that leads to cytoskeletal disintegration.

Within 24 hours of injury, a single axon produces multiple axonal sprouts. At the tip of these sprouts, a growth cone exists that has an affinity for the fibronectin and laminin of the Schwann cell basal lamina. The growth cone explores the distal environment for an appropriate physical substrate (Fig. 16).

The inflammatory response in wallerian degeneration

Macrophages, T cells, and neutrophils infiltrate the site of an injury within 2 days. There are 2 populations of macrophages in an injured peripheral nerve: resident and recruited. Resident endoneurial macrophages constitute approximately 4% of the endoneurial cell population and respond extremely rapidly to injury. They are joined by recruited macrophages from the vascular supply attracted by locally produced chemokines. These macrophages penetrate the tubes of the Schwann cell, degrade the myelin sheaths, and phagocytose the axonal debris that occurs with degeneration (see Fig. 16). Schwann cells may participate in the breakdown of myelin if the numbers of macrophages are depleted. Although the endoneurium and basal lamina remain intact, the neural tube eventually collapses as the myelin and axonal contents are digested. The process continues until

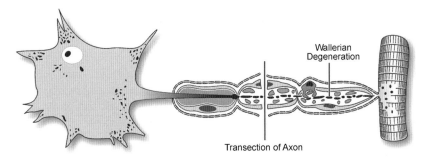

Fig. 15. Transection injury such as could occur with a scalpel or straight fissure bur and accompanying axonal degeneration, resulting in dissolution of distal myelin sheaths, degeneration of axoplasm distally, and sealing of the tip of the proximal stump of the axon. (*Courtesy of* Don Johnson, Emory University, Atlanta, GA.)

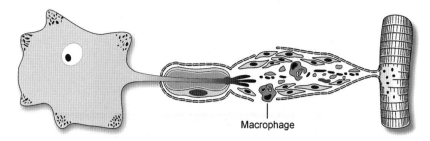

Fig. 16. The inflammatory response. The Schwann cell tube is invaded by macrophages that breach the basal lamina. Schwann cells distal to the injury site proliferate and axon sprouts begin to emerge from the proximal stump. (*Courtesy of* Don Johnson, Emory University, Atlanta, GA.)

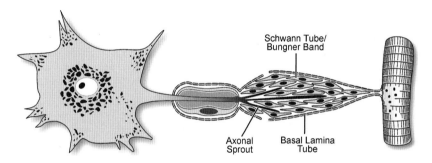

Fig. 17. Axonal regeneration: the proliferating Schwann cells form a tube (also known as the band of Bungner). Axon sprouts form from the proximal end of the axon. (*Courtesy of* Don Johnson, Emory University, Atlanta, GA.)

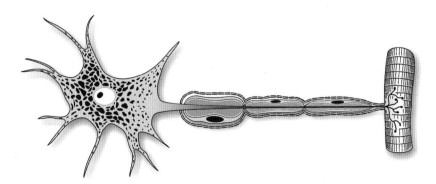

Fig. 18. Daughter Schwann Cells and complete regeneration in a less than critical nerve gap. Daughter Schwann cells remyelinate the regenerating axon. The new myelin sheaths are thinner and the intermodal distances are shorter than the more proximal counterparts of the axon. (*Courtesy of* Don Johnson, Emory University, Atlanta, GA.)

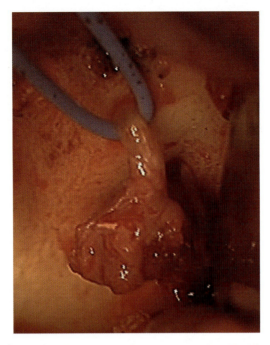

Fig. 19. Neuroma of the peripheral trigeminal nerve at its exit from the right mental foramen.

the neural components of the axons are completely resorbed, at which time the neural tube becomes replaced by Schwann cells and macrophages.

Schwann cells and axonal regeneration

By 3 to 4 days after injury, Schwann cells throughout the distal stump and at the tip of the proximal stump start to divide. The proliferating Schwann cells then organize into columns and form the bands of Bungner, which are arrays of Schwann cells within a space circumscribed by the basal lamina (Schwann tube) (Fig. 17). The spouts from the proximal stump of the axon grow toward the lesion site within the basal lamina tubes that enveloped their parent axons. With successful elongation, and in the case of minimal separation of the 2 ends of the damaged axon, there may be no axonal misrouting, and remyelination of the axon from the daughter Schwann cells will take place (Fig. 18).

Pathway selection

If axons degenerate without rupture of the basal lamina that surrounds each Schwann tube, the axon sprouts are less likely to be misrouted. In traumatic injuries to the peripheral nerve resulting in complete disruption, the nerve ends become a swollen mass of disorganized Schwann cells, capillaries, fibroblasts, macrophages, and collagen fibers. Regenerating axons reach the swollen bulb of the proximal stump and encounter significant barriers to further regeneration. Most sprouts will remain in the endoneurium, but others may traverse into the epineurium through breaches in the damaged perineurium, or may grow ectopically between the layers of the perineurium. In both situations, their behavior may produce a painful neuroma (Fig. 19).

Summary

Oral and maxillofacial surgeons caring for patients who have sustained a nerve injury to a branch of the peripheral trigeminal nerve must possess a basic understanding of the response of the peripheral nerves to trauma. The series of events that subsequently take place are largely dependent on the injury type and severity. Regeneration of the peripheral nerve is possible in many instances and future manipulation of the regenerative microenvironment will lead to advances in the management of these difficult injuries.

Further readings

Burnett MG, Zager EL. Pathophysiology of peripheral nerve injury: a brief review. Neurosurg Focus 2004;16:E1.
Hall S. The response to injury in the peripheral nervous system. J Bone Joint Surg Br 2005;87(10):1309–19.
Lundborg G. Nerve injury and repair. Regeneration, reconstruction and cortical re-modeling. 2nd edition. Philadelphia: Elsevier; 2004.
Maggi SP, Lowe JB, Mackinnon SE. Pathophysiology of nerve injury. Clin Plast Surg 2003;30:109–26.
Seddon JJ. Three types of nerve injury. Brain 1943;66:237.
Sunderland S. A classification of peripheral nerve injuries produced by loss of function. Brain 1951;74:491.

Clinical Evaluation of Peripheral Trigeminal Nerve Injuries

Roger A. Meyer, DDS, MS, MD[a,*], Shahrokh C. Bagheri, DMD, MD[b,c,d,e]

[a]Maxillofacial Consultations Ltd, 1021 Holt's Ferry, Greensboro, GA 30642, USA
[b]Private Practice, Georgia Oral & Facial Surgery, 1880 West Oak Parkway, Suite 215, Marietta, GA 30062, USA
[c]Division of Oral & Maxillofacial Surgery, Department of Surgery, Northside Hospital, 1000 Johnson Ferry Road, Atlanta, GA 30342, USA
[d]Department of Surgery, School of Medicine, Emory University, 1365 Clifton Road NE, Atlanta, GA 30322, USA
[e]Department of Oral & Maxillofacial Surgery, School of Dentistry, Medical College of Georgia, 1120 15th Street, Augusta, GA 30912, USA

The purpose of evaluation of a patient with a sensory nerve injury is to obtain information about the circumstances of the injury and its subsequent course, perform an examination of the area containing the sensory dysfunction, complete a series of testing maneuvers that will outline the area of sensory deficit, quantify the magnitude and character of the deficit, and record it in an objective manner that can be used as a basis for comparison with serial examinations, if needed. Accurate and complete records of the evaluation are essential, because they may be important in making decisions regarding treatment of the nerve injury. Good medical records may be helpful in the case of legal action, and they are indispensable in retrospective studies of patient care.

To the clinician inexperienced in the management of sensory nerve injuries in the oral and maxillofacial regions, evaluation of a patient who has sustained an injury to one of the peripheral branches of the trigeminal nerve can be a frustrating or intimidating encounter. Although there are many advanced, sophisticated, and technologically involved methods for evaluating nerve function that are used primarily in laboratory and clinical studies by researchers, the clinical evaluation of an injured sensory nerve can be accurately and adequately done by the simple, straightforward evaluation presented in this article. Such evaluation can be completed by any clinician in less than 30 minutes for most patients. In the authors' practice, a printed form is completed by the patient before being seen by the clinician, and this provides much essential information about the patient's complaints, progress of symptoms and their severity, and effect on orofacial function. Various aspects of this form are presented and discussed. The results of the evaluation are easily interpreted, regardless of whether or not the clinician has microneurosurgical skills. In the case of a nonmicrosurgeon, information gained from the nerve injury evaluation will enable the clinician to make an appropriate decision regarding referral for further evaluation and/or possible microsurgical repair of a nerve injury. Alternative methods of nerve evaluation are discussed and can be perused further by the reader by consulting the references listed in Further readings.

The essential elements of the evaluation of the patient with a peripheral sensory nerve injury include the history; the general head, neck, and oral examination; neurosensory testing; imaging studies; diagnosis; and classification of the nerve injury. Each of these is discussed in this article.

History

The history of a peripheral trigeminal sensory nerve injury begins with the patient's chief complaint, or the reason that brought the patient to your attention. It is generally one of decreased

* Corresponding author.
E-mail address: rameyer@aol.com

or altered sensation (paresthesia), or of painful or unpleasant sensation (dysesthesia). It is important to distinguish between these 2 types of sensory dysfunction because the clinical examination of each is different (see later discussion). Some patients may complain of paresthesia and dysesthesia. Patients often have difficulty expressing themselves with regard to sensory symptoms, so the exact nature of their affliction may be better determined by having the patient complete a printed questionnaire before being seen for evaluation by the clinician (Box 1).

The patient who complains of decreased or altered sensation may state the problem as numbness. However, this is merely a lay term that requires clarification to be meaningful in the clinical sense. The patient who complains of numbness may be implying a level of altered sensation anywhere along a spectrum from minimal sensory loss to total loss of sensation, as well as some component of dysesthesia. To assist the patient in describing the nature of the sensory dysfunction, it is helpful to include a list of descriptive words on the printed form that the patient completes before being seen by the clinician (Box 2). Patients may or may not complain of interference with everyday orofacial activities because of numbness. However, several functions, including speech, chewing food, and playing of wind musical instruments, are frequently found to be compromised when there is decreased or lost sensation.

Patients who experience a painful or unpleasant sensation are asked whether it is constant or intermittent. Constant pain is usually seen in patients with long-term well-established dysesthesia. There is frequently a central component as well as that caused by the injured peripheral nerve. For instance, central pain may develop in time secondary to the loss of afferent input to the central nervous system (CNS) from the periphery, so-called deafferentation, caused by failure of transmission of the injured nerve. If the pain is intermittent, it may be spontaneous or stimulus induced. Spontaneous pain may be of brief duration (seconds) or longer (minutes to hours, or constant). Stimulus-induced pain is characteristically brief (seconds), and it is usually associated with the performance of a common, everyday maneuver by the patient. Such pain is usually described by the patient as hypersensitivity (Box 3). The intensity or severity of the pain may be estimated by having the patient select descriptive words from a written list (see Box 2) or use a visual analog scale (VAS), in which 0 indicates no pain and 10 implies the worst pain the patient has ever experienced (Box 4). The amount of estimated impairment of orofacial functions in either the patient with decreased altered sensation or unpleasant sensation is determined by having the patient complete the printed form shown in Box 5.

Patients who have sustained a lingual nerve injury often complain of altered taste sensation (parageusia). The degree of taste impairment is estimated by the patient as part of the history of the present illness (see Box 5). Rarely, if ever, is altered taste the chief complaint of a patient with a lingual nerve injury.

The patient is asked whether there is anything that has relieved the pain (medications, application of heat or cold, rest, and so forth). In some patients with pain of long duration, there is a history of

---

Box 1. The chief complaint. In the printed form used in the authors' practice, the patient is asked to supply information that accurately describes the reason for the visit

Do you have altered, abnormal, or absent sensation (feeling) in your face, mouth, jaws, or neck? (Circle all that apply):

Right   Left   Both sides

forehead   eyebrow   cheek   ear   nose
mouth   upper lip   upper gums   palate   upper teeth
lower lip lower gums tongue   chin   neck

other _____

What is your **most** distressing symptom? (Circle)

LOSS OF FEELING (numbness) PAIN or BOTH (pain and numbness)

> **Box 2. Words helpful to patients in describing their sensory dysfunction**
>
> a) Which of the following words (symptoms) best describe(s) your complaint of **numbness**? (Circle all that apply; add any others you think are pertinent to your condition.)
>
> | | | | | |
> |---|---|---|---|---|
> | numb | wet | stretched | vibrating | others: |
> | tickling | rubbery | swollen | drawing | |
> | tingling | cool | tight | pulling | |
> | twitching | warm | wooden | itching | |
>
> b) Which of the following best describe(s) your complaint of **pain**? (Circle all that apply; add any others you think describe your condition.)
>
> | | | | |
> |---|---|---|---|
> | hot | pricking | electric shock | constant |
> | cold | stinging | agonizing | intermittent |
> | tender | burning | excruciating | |
> | sore | painful | | others: |

misuse or abuse of medications, and the patient may request prescription medications on the first visit. In most cases, this is inappropriate and should not be provided. Consultation with all the patient's other practitioners may reveal multiple inappropriate prescriptions for medications with high addictive potential.

The history of the present illness includes the incident or operation (eg, lower third molar removal, mandibular osteotomy, placement of dental implant, maxillofacial fracture) that preceded the onset of the chief complaint, the date of its occurrence, the symptoms, and their progress or change in the time since onset, and any perceived orofacial functional impairments of which the patient complains. This information can best be determined by asking the following preliminary screening questions: (1) What happened to initiate the onset of your symptoms? (2) When (date) did it happen? (3) When did your primary symptom (numbness and/or pain) begin? (4) What is the progress or change in your symptom(s) since onset (getting worse, getting better, staying the same)? (Box 6).

> **Box 3. Daily orofacial activities associated with onset of intermittent pain**
>
> Circle any of the following stimuli that cause your pain:
>
> | | | |
> |---|---|---|
> | touch | brushing teeth | drinking liquids |
> | washing | smoking | speaking |
> | shaving | kissing | swallowing |
> | chewing food | placing make up | smiling |
>
> others _____
>
> After any of the above stimuli, how long does your pain last?
>
> seconds   minutes   hours   days
>
> Does anything relieve your pain?   (Circle) YES   NO
>
> If YES, what? _____

> **Box 4. The VAS assists the patient in determining the severity of pain**
>
> On the scale shown, if 0 represents no pain and 10 represents the worst pain imaginable, circle the number that represents your typical level of pain:
>
> ```
> 0   1   2   3   4   5   6   7   8   9   10
> No                                       Worst
> pain                                     pain
> ```

The incident or operation that initiated the onset of sensory symptoms is often helpful in locating the site of nerve injury. For example, if, after removal of the mandibular right third molar, a patient complains of right tongue numbness, there has most likely been an injury to the right lingual nerve (LN) in its location on the medial surface of the right mandible adjacent to the site of tooth removal; the patient who complains of right lower lip and chin numbness probably sustained an injury to the right inferior alveolar nerve (IAN) adjacent to the third molar socket. If, after a facial fracture involving the left inferior orbital rim, the patient complains of left midfacial and upper lip numbness, most likely the left infraorbital nerve (IFN) has been injured within the inferior orbital canal at or near its exit from the left infraorbital foramen. Sensory changes in the lower lip or chin following placement of dental implants are generally caused by direct contact of the IAN or mental nerve (MN) with a drill or the implant itself. Special notice is taken of the patient whose onset of altered sensation is without an associated incident or injury. Such a patient requires the evaluation presented here to rule out the presence of problems in the oral and maxillofacial regions. Failing to find a cause there,

> **Box 5. Orofacial functional impairment. Assessment of interference of sensory dysfunction with the performance of common, everyday activities**
>
> Are you currently experiencing any of the following impairments because of your nerve injury? Check (x) any that apply to you and note the level of impairment (1, 2, or 3) as follows:
> 1 = minimal interference with normal performance of this activity;
> 2 = moderate (50%) interference; 3 = total or nearly total interference
>
> Impairment level (1, 2, or 3)
> _____ ( ) Lip, cheek, or tongue biting (circle)
> _____ ( ) Burning of the lip or tongue with hot fluids/food
> _____ ( ) Dribbling of food, drooling of liquids/saliva
> _____ ( ) Difficulty chewing food
> _____ ( ) Difficulty swallowing
> _____ ( ) Lost, decreased, or altered taste sensation
> _____ ( ) Difficulty speaking
> _____ ( ) Difficulty with toothbrushing, using dental floss
> _____ ( ) Difficulty applying lipstick, makeup
> _____ ( ) Difficulty sleeping
> _____ ( ) Difficulty playing wind musical instruments
> _____ ( ) Difficulty performing work duties
> _____ ( ) Interference with relationship with spouse or other
> _____ ( ) Other: _____

> **Box 6. Important information in the history of nerve injury (history of present illness)**
>
> When did your symptoms begin? (date) _____
>
> Was there dental or surgical treatment or an injury associated with the onset of your symptoms?   YES   NO
>
> If yes, please indicate (x) what was done or what happened and when:
>
>   date
> ( ) Local anesthetic injections for dental work . . . . . . _____
> ( ) Removal of impacted teeth . . . . _____
> ( ) Osteotomy (surgery for jaw deformity) . . . . _____
> ( ) Dental implants . . . . _____
> ( ) Root canal filling . . . . _____
> ( ) Facial or jaw fracture . . . . _____
> ( ) Other   . . . . _____
>
> Name of surgeon or dentist _____
> Address (street, city, state) _____
> _____
>
> Telephone (area code) _____ (number) _____
>
> Since the onset of your symptoms, what change has occurred in their intensity (numbness), frequency, and/or severity (pain)?
>
> (check [x] which):
>
> ( ) No change
> ( ) Minimal improvement of numbness and/or decrease in pain
> ( ) Moderate improvement
> ( ) Marked improvement
> ( ) Minimal worsening of pain and/or increase in numbness
> ( ) Moderate worsening
> ( ) Marked worsening

the patient should be referred to a neurologist for further evaluation of a central cause (tumor, vascular anomaly, infection, metabolic disorder, and so forth).

The date of the incident or onset of sensory changes is important because there is a timetable for the pathophysiologic response of a peripheral nerve to injury (Wallerian degeneration). In time, the axons distal to the injury site undergo necrosis and phagocytosis. Repair is attempted by outgrowth of axonal sprouts from the proximal nerve stump. If the distal nerve is not spontaneously recannulated by new axons within a critical period of time, its superstructure is replaced by scar tissue and becomes incapable of repair, either spontaneously or by surgical intervention. There is a well-known window of opportunity of approximately 6 months from the time of injury when surgical repair of a nerve gives the best chance of a favorable result. After that, success rates decrease greatly with each passing month until a critical mass of distal nerve tissue is replaced by scar and is no longer capable of repair. In humans, this time has been estimated to be between 9 and 15 months, depending on the age and general health of the patient, and other individual characteristics not yet fully appreciated. Therefore, it behooves the clinician who initially evaluates the patient with a sensory nerve injury to note the date of the injury as accurately as possible, so that surgical intervention that might be indicated for a nerve injury that is not resolving spontaneously can be done in a timely fashion.

Numbness or painful sensations may not begin at the same time as the incident or operation associated with the nerve injury. For instance, seepage of root canal medicaments from the tooth apex following an endodontic procedure may take 1 or more days to reach the adjacent inferior alveolar canal (IAC) and cause a chemical burn of the IAN. Or, after bone preparation for dental implant placement, edema secondary to heat generated by the drill may develop slowly with delayed compression of the IAN and the onset of lower lip numbness and pain not noted by the patient for up to 24 hours after the procedure. If the IAN is not directly injured but the bony wall of the IAC is disrupted during elevation and removal of a mandibular third molar, excessive bone may be regenerated during the healing process, causing narrowing of the canal diameter and delayed compression of the IAN from 1 to several months after tooth removal. Such examples serve to explain why, although most sensory nerve injuries result in immediate onset of symptoms, onset of sensory dysfunction is delayed in some patients.

The progress of sensory symptoms is important because, in a period of days, weeks, or months following the nerve injury, the patient may show improvement or deterioration in sensory status or undergo no change. The patient may also exhibit these changes in a period of repeated evaluations. In patients who are improving, an expectant course is followed, in which serial evaluations are done at regular intervals (weekly, biweekly, or monthly) as long as they continue to show documented subjective and objective improvement at each subsequent visit. A patient who fails to show improvement of neurosensory status from one evaluation to the next will not resume improvement sometime in the future. Therefore, this patient has reached a plateau, and a decision regarding surgical intervention should be considered at that time, rather than following the patient further in the vain hope of resumption of improvement. Whether or not a patient is improving is based not only on subjective information (the patient's history) but also on objective evidence (discussed later). In the course of recovery from a sensory nerve injury, new symptoms may occur. Most commonly, persistent numbness is the patient's first complaint. Although pain may be present initially as well, it often develops days or weeks later, and it may increase in frequency and duration, become episodic or constant, and be spontaneous or associated with orofacial maneuvers (discussed earlier).

Equipment

The well-equipped clinician's office should already contain the instruments and supplies needed for examination of the patient with a sensory nerve injury. Sterile gloves, cotton swabs, tongue blades, or mouth mirror and calipers, as well as local anesthetic needles, carpules, and syringes are sufficient for most patients (Fig. 1). A vitalometer (pulp tester) is sometimes helpful as an alternative method of assessing response to pain.

Head, neck, and oral examination

An examination is completed on all patients to include eyes, ears, nose, face, temporomandibular joints, neck, oral cavity, and pharynx. The components of the screening examination specific for the patient with sensory nerve injury are outlined in Fig. 2. The first step is inspection. On the patient who

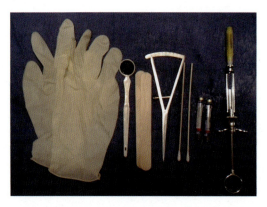

Fig. 1. Equipment used in examination of the patient with a sensory nerve injury includes (left to right) gloves, mouth mirror, tongue blades, calipers, cotton swabs, local anesthetic carpules, syringe, and 27-gauge needle.

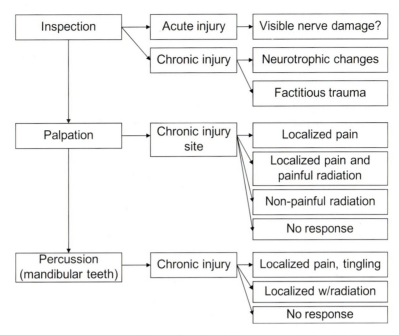

Fig. 2. Important components of screening examination for patient with sensory nerve injury. Details are provided in the text.

has sustained acute trauma, the examiner looks for evidence of an acute injury (missile wound, laceration, facial bone fracture, other trauma). A nerve transsection, avulsion, partial tear, compression, or crushing may be able to be directly visualized through a wound or laceration. In other patients, the clinician looks for evidence of recent or past injury or surgery (eg, lacerations or incisions, or scars from previous wounds), or neurotrophic changes of the skin (edema, erythema, ulcerations, hypohydrosis, loss of hair, hypokeratosis) that may occur following sensory loss in that area. The patient with long-standing sensory nerve dysfunction may subject the affected soft tissues to repeated factitious (self-induced) habits (Fig. 3). In the neck, scars from past injury or incision in response to stimulation (gentle stroking with the examining finger or a cotton swab) may exhibit symptoms and signs of sympathetic nervous system hyperactivity (hyperesthesia, sweating, blanching, flushing, skin temperature changes) in the skin area supplied by the injured nerve. Such signs may indicate so-called sympathetic-mediated pain (SMP; also known as reflex sympathetic dystrophy [RSD]) (Fig. 4).

Palpation or percussion directly over the accessible area of the LN (on the medial surface of the mandible adjacent to the third molar), the MN (over the mental foramen, usually located between the apices of the mandibular premolar teeth) or the IFN (located just below the midportion of the inferior orbital rim) may induce 1 of 3 sensory responses, each called a trigger (Fig. 5). First, a painful, electric shock sensation may be evoked that is limited to the area of palpation. Second, the sensation may

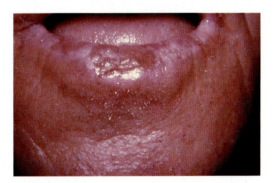

Fig. 3. An example of factitious injury in a dennervated area with neurotrophic changes. A 54-year-old man was referred for treatment of suspected malignancy of lower lip. History revealed loss of sensation to entire lower lip and chin after sustaining bilateral mandibular fractures 10 years previously. Patient had developed a habit of chewing the numb lower lip. Multiple biopsies of lower lip revealed only acute and chronic inflammation without evidence of dysplasia or malignancy.

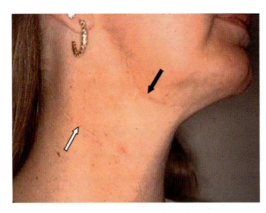

Fig. 4. 40-year-old woman with right neck scars from previous surgery (*white and black arrows*). Patient developed constant burning pain and, in response to gentle stroking of the submandibular scar (*black arrow*) with a cotton swab, she complained of bursts of additional severe pain, the scar became reddened, and the surrounding area exhibited sweating and blanching. Abolition of pain and physical manifestations by administration of a local anesthetic block of the ipsilateral stellate ganglion confirmed the diagnosis of sympathetic-mediated pain (RSD).

radiate distally into the area supplied by the nerve (eg, palpation of the lingual nerve causes painful sensations in the ipsilateral floor of the mouth and tongue). Third, nonpainful sensations (tingling, crawling, itching) may radiate from the area of nerve palpation. In some patients, palpation of the injured nerve produces no trigger response. In most patients, based on the authors' subsequent direct observation during microsurgical repair of the nerve, a trigger area denotes the site of the nerve injury. A painful response without radiation often indicates a complete nerve transection with

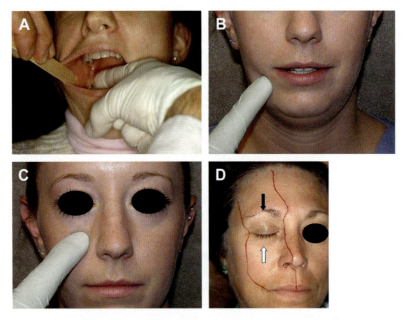

Fig. 5. Palpation over an area of suspected nerve injury may elicit a trigger response, with or without radiation distally into the tissues supplied by the nerve. (*A*) Examiner's finger is palpating the soft tissues on lingual aspect of previously removed mandibular third molar to check for trigger response from injury site of right LN. (*B*) Palpating skin over mental foramen may elicit trigger response from underlying injured MN. Palpation can also be done intraorally in the mandibular buccal vestibule between the first and second premolar teeth. (*C*) Just below the inferior orbital rim, palpation of an injured IFN is done to check for a trigger response. This area can be palpated in some patients intraorally in the maxillary buccal vestibule above the root apices of the first and second premolars. (*D*) This patient sustained multiple facial injuries including superior and inferior orbital rim fractures. She complained of right facial and forehead numbness and stimulus-evoked pain (allodynia). The pain was reproduced on examination by palpation over the right supraorbital (*black arrow*) and infraorbital (*white arrow*) foramina (trigger areas), and it was abolished by local anesthetic blocks of the supraorbital nerve and IFN. At surgery, both nerves were found to have neuromas-in-continuity. After excision of neuromas and neurorrhaphies, the patient regained useful sensory function and experienced lasting relief of pain.

a proximal stump neuroma, whereas a painful response or a nonpainful response with radiation is a sign of a partial nerve transection or a neuroma-in-continuity. In some cases with complete nerve transection, there are radiating sensations from the trigger area that probably represent phantom pain. Occasionally, patients with significant nerve injuries fail to give a trigger response to palpation over the injury site. Therefore, a trigger response should be considered good evidence of a significant nerve injury, whereas a lack of response does not rule out the presence of injury.

Percussion of the mandibular teeth may cause painful or tingling sensations that may or may not radiate into the lower lip or chin. Palpation or gentle stroking of the lower lip or chin may likewise produce sensations in the lower teeth. The significance of these findings in relation to the type of injury of the IAN is not well understood, because the findings at surgery do not seem to show a consistent relationship of the severity of the injury with the results of examination. Vitalometer testing of the mandibular teeth provides additional information about the function of the IAN, similar to that of level C testing (discussed later).

Objective testing of taste function is a detailed, technically demanding endeavor, and it is not included as part of the routine clinical examination of the patient with nerve injury. After nerve lingual repair, the patient is routinely questioned about the status of taste sensation as part of the follow-up visits. The degree of return of taste sensation after successful recovery of general sensation to the tongue and associated tissues is difficult to predict, and it does not always equal that of general sensory function. The chorda tympani fibers that conduct taste impulses, although traveling with the LN, have their cell bodies in the facial (seventh cranial) nerve nucleus. These cell bodies show less potential for recovery after injury than do the general sensory cell bodies of the trigeminal nerve. The patient who complains of altered taste sensation is advised of the possibility of persistence of some degree of parageusia, whether or not the LN is surgically repaired.

Neurosensory testing

Neurosensory testing (NST) includes a group of standardized maneuvers designed to evaluate sensory function as objectively as possible within the clinical setting. The patient is seated comfortably, and all tests are administered with the patient's eyes closed. When the patient's lips are being tested, they should be separated so that pressure or vibration of applied stimuli is not transmitted to the opposite lip. The examiner explains each maneuver beforehand with reassurance that the stimuli will be applied gently and with due concern for any areas of pain or hypersensitivity that the patient may have described in the history. The contralateral normal side is always tested first to determine the patient's control responses.

The examiner begins by determining the area of altered sensation by using the marching needle technique in which a 27-gauge needle is advanced from an adjacent normal area to the area of sensory dysfunction as indicated by the patient in the history. The needle touches the surface mucosa or skin lightly at 1- to 2-mm intervals until the patient indicates (by raising the ipsilateral hand) the point at which the sensation of the needle begins to change. This process is repeated until the border of the entire area of altered sensation is outlined. The area may be indicated by marking the skin with a marking pen that can later be easily removed with alcohol or orange solvent (Fig. 6). Further NST is then performed, first on the contralateral normal side (for example, the left lower lip, to establish normal responses for that patient) and then on the ipsilateral side (for example, the right lower lip with altered sensation, to ascertain the level of abnormal responses). In case of bilateral nerve injuries, an adjacent normal area is used for control responses (eg, for bilateral IAN injuries, the normal vermilion border of the upper lip for comparison with bilateral lower lip numbness and the adjacent cheek or submental area for bilateral chin numbness; for bilateral IFN injuries, the normal lower lip vermilion border for comparison with bilateral upper lip numbness; for bilateral LN injuries, the normal lower labial mucosa for comparison with bilateral tongue and lingual gingival numbness).

When performing NST, it is helpful to understand the concept of threshold of response. When a stimulus (ie, a needle) is applied to the skin or mucosal surface, it is done initially with little or no pressure exerted and with no indentation of the surface tissue. If the patient feels the stimulus, it is noted that the response was at the normal threshold. If the patient does not respond to the stimulus, then the stimulus is applied again with just enough pressure to cause indentation, but not piercing of the skin or mucosa. If the patient now feels the stimulus, the response was at an increased threshold.

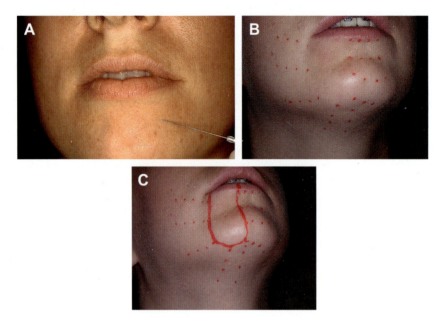

Fig. 6. Determining the boundaries of the area of altered sensation from an injury to the IAN on the patient's right lower lip and chin. (*A*) (*Left*) The 27-gauge needle is advanced (the marching needle) in stepwise fashion with multiple light contact points starting from an area of normal sensation on the left chin until the patient indicates a change or loss of sensation. (*B*) (*Right*) The needle contact is made on multiple spots (indicated by red dots) to complete the outline of the border of the area of altered sensation. (*C*) (*Below*) The area of altered sensation of the right lower lip and chin is outlined with an erasable marking pen.

This result indicates a nerve that has sustained injury but still retains the ability to transmit electrical impulses from the periphery to the CNS, albeit compromised in the number of axons able to transmit and/or their speed of transmission (Fig. 7). If the patient still does not respond at the increased threshold, no additional pressure is placed and the patient is said to have no response. If the patient does not respond to a stimulus applied at increased threshold, there will be no response to further pressure applied by the stimulus. To further increase the pressure applied to the stimulus (needle) at this point will cause penetration of the mucosa or skin with attendant bleeding, and add no useful information. This concept allows a simple, but accurate, measurement of responses to static light touch and painful stimuli (level B and level C testing are discussed later), and provides an acceptable substitute for more elaborate, sophisticated, and expensive testing modalities.

The examination of the patient with decreased altered sensation differs from that of the patient with unpleasant altered sensation because the goals for diagnosis and treatment are not the same for these 2 categories of patients. In the former (decreased altered sensation), the aim is to improve or

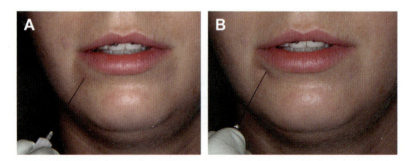

Fig. 7. Determining the pressure threshold required to elicit a response to an applied stimulus. (*A*) (*Left*) The stimulus (27-gauge needle) is applied lightly without indentation of the skin. If the patient indicates that the stimulus was felt, this is a response at the normal threshold. (*B*) (*Right*) If the patient does not feel a stimulus applied at the normal threshold of pressure, a second stimulus is applied with just enough additional pressure to indent (but not pierce) the skin. If the patient indicates that this stimulus was felt, this is a response at an increased threshold (abnormal response). See text for further explanation.

restore sensation, whereas, in the latter, relief or reduction of pain is the primary objective. Therefore, the examination of each of these 2 types of patients is described separately.

Decreased Altered Sensation

Three levels of testing are done on the patient with decreased or altered sensation without pain. The goal of NST for this type of patient is to grade the level of impairment of sensory function as normal, or mild, moderate, or severe hypoesthesia, or complete (ie, anesthesia). The tests are done in order and one level of testing may or may not lead to another, depending on the patient's responses (Fig. 8).

Level A testing includes evaluation of directional discrimination (moving stimuli), 2-point discrimination (2pd), and stimulus localization, which measure function of larger-diameter, well-myelinated a and b fibers (5–12 μm diameter). Directional discrimination is evaluated by lightly applying a series of 10 randomly directed moving strokes (skin only) with a cotton swab (or a soft camel hair brush) to the test area (normal side always first). The strokes are directed horizontally, vertically, or diagonally (Fig. 9). After each stroke, the patient is asked to indicate the direction verbally or retrace it with a cotton swab. The normal response on the control side is 9 or 10 out of 10 correct direction identifications. Eight or fewer correct identifications on the abnormal side indicate the level of impairment, which is recorded as 7/10, 3/10, 1/10, and so forth.

Determination of 2pd is done with calipers (or cotton pliers and a millimeter ruler) (Fig. 10). This test is begun with the points of the calipers together (zero distance). As contact is gently made with the calipers, the patient is asked to identify (verbally or with fingers) whether contact is made with 1 point or 2 points. The distance between the caliper tips is increased by 1 mm for each subsequent application until the patient is able to identify 2 simultaneous points of contact (threshold distance). Further applications are made to overshoot this distance by 2 to 3 mm, then the process is reversed from that point in 1-mm increments until the patient again no longer perceives simultaneous contact with 2 points. Generally, in both the ascending and descending distances, the threshold is the same or within 1 mm. Occasionally, the examiner will apply only 1 caliper tip to verify that the patient is not trying to game the system. Normal values for 2pd are given in Table 1. Alternative level A testing armamentaria include the Disk-Criminator and the 2-point pressure esthesiometer.

Stimulus localization is a method of estimating the amount of synthesia (the inability to determine the exact point of application, nature [sharp, dull], and size [surface area] of a discrete stimulus), which is often associated with partial sensory loss or with a recovering sensory nerve injury. This estimation is easily done by lightly contacting the skin with the wooden end of a cotton swab stick,

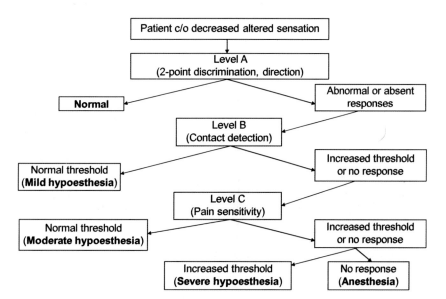

Fig. 8. The steps in NST for evaluating a patient with nerve injury with decreased altered sensation. Diagnoses are in bold type. See text for further discussion.

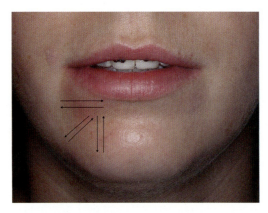

Fig. 9. Directional discrimination (moving brush stroke direction identification): the thin black arrows indicate horizontal, vertical, or diagonal directions of the strokes that are applied randomly by the examiner. After each application, the patient is asked to duplicate the direction of the stroke with a cotton swab.

and then asking the patient to touch the same spot with another swab stick. A normal patient response is contact within 1 to 2 mm of the examiner's contact point. Generally, 5 contacts are applied in each test area (Fig. 11).

Patients who give responses within the normal range to level A testing in the area of altered sensation are judged to be normal, and no further testing is necessary. The patient who gives abnormal or no responses is impaired and the examiner proceeds with level B testing.

Level B testing evaluates responses to non-noxious stimuli (ie, static light touch), which assesses the function of smaller a and b fibers (4–8 μm). The test area is touched lightly without indentation with the wooden end of a cotton swab stick. The patient is asked to raise the ipsilateral hand when contact is felt. Response to contact without skin indentation is at the normal threshold, and no further NST is necessary for this patient. If the patient fails to respond, the stimulus is repeated, but this time with sufficient pressure to cause indentation. If the patient now responds to the contact, this is at an increased threshold, and this is an abnormal response. As a third alternative, the patient may still not respond at the increased threshold. Patients who respond at an increased threshold or give no response proceed to level C testing. Alternative level B testing can be done using Semmes-Weinstein monofilaments (Fig. 12).

Level C testing measures response to noxious stimuli. These impulses are carried by scantily myelinated or nonmyelinated smallest diameter c fibers (0.05–1.0 μm). The test area is contacted without indentation with the tip of a 27-guage needle. The normal response is that the patient raises the ipsilateral hand when contact is felt. If the patient gives no response, the test area is slightly indented (but not pierced) by the needle tip. If the patient now responds, this is at an increased threshold, which is an abnormal response. If the patient fails to respond at the increased threshold, no further increase in pressure is applied to the needle tip, and the patient is judged nonresponsive.

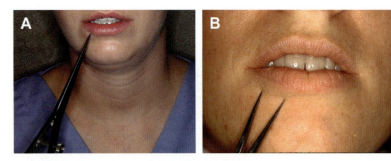

Fig. 10. Level A testing for 2-point discrimination. (*A*) (*Left*) Measurement is begun by contact with the calipers closed together. (*B*) (*Right*) With each succeeding contact, the caliper beaks are separated by 1 additional millimeter until the patient indicates that 2 simultaneously applied contact points are felt (at 5 mm in this patient).

Table 1
Normal values for static 2pd

Test area	Average normal threshold distance (mm)[a]	Upper normal limit (mm)[b]
Forehead	13.0	22.0
Cheek (hairy)	9.0	17.0
Upper lip (skin)	4.5	8.0
Upper lip (mucosal)	3.0	6.0
Lower lip (mucosal)	3.5	6.5
Lower lip (skin)	5.0	9.0
Chin	9.0	18.0
Tongue (tip)	3.0	4.5
Tongue (dorsum)	5.0	12.0

[a] Values determined from the literature.
[b] Distance greater than this is considered abnormal.

Alternative testing methods include an algometer, thermal discs, and a vitalometer (pulp tester) (Fig. 13).

Depending on responses to level A, B, and C testing, the patient who is evaluated for decreased altered sensation may be diagnosed as normal, mild hypoesthesia, moderate hypoesthesia, severe hypoesthesia, or anesthesia, as outlined in Fig. 8.

If the patient has sustained acute maxillofacial trauma and is conscious and cooperative, level B and level C NST is done to screen for an injury to 1 or more of the peripheral branches of the trigeminal nerve, which are frequently involved in fractures or lacerations. Having this information before the patient is taken to the operating room may modify the surgical approach, and it is a useful baseline for further follow-up, whether the injured nerve is repaired at the same time as the other facial injuries or at some later date.

Unpleasant Altered Sensation

Three levels of NST are done on the patient with painful sensation, but the tests and their goals differ from those of the patient with decreased sensation (Fig. 14). In contrast with the patient with decreased sensation, all levels of testing are done in the patient with painful sensation, regardless of response at each level. The aims of these tests are to elicit and characterize the types of abnormal painful responses to various stimuli (hyperesthesia), which may have implications for treatment and prognosis.

Level A testing for the patient with unpleasant or painful sensations determines whether an innocuous mechanical stimulus (not normally painful) evokes a pain response within the distribution of the injured nerve. The test is given by applying a gentle stroke with a cotton swab or camel hair brush to the skin or mucosal surface of the normal contralateral side first as control, then repeating the maneuver within the abnormal area. Pain in response to a stimulus that is not normally painful and that ceases when the stimulus is withdrawn is termed allodynia, and is frequently described by the patient as hypersensitive. The duration and intensity (patient's description or VAS) of the evoked pain are noted.

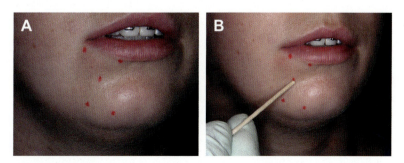

Fig. 11. Level A testing for stimulus localization. (*A*) Five standard contact points (*red dots*) for stimulus localization. (*B*) The examiner contacts the patients skin lightly (no skin indentation) with a cotton swab at each contact point. After each contact by the examiner, the patient is asked to contact exactly the same point.

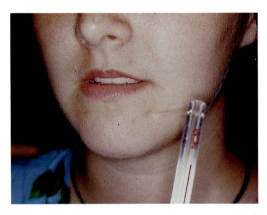

Fig. 12. Semmes-Weinstein monofilament is an alternative method of evaluating static light touch (level B testing) also used in clinical and laboratory research.

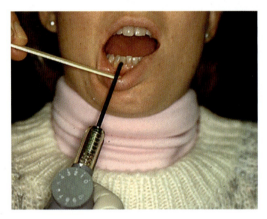

Fig. 13. Vitalometer readings of the lower teeth can be used as another method of level C testing for response to painful stimuli.

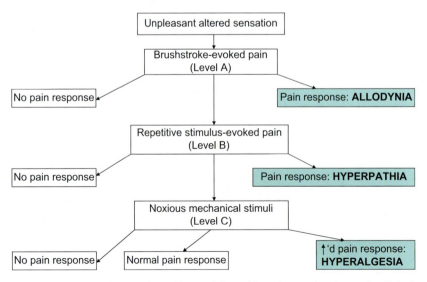

Fig. 14. The steps in NST for evaluating a patient with nerve injury with unpleasant altered sensation. Pain diagnoses are in bold type. See text for further discussion.

The goal of level B testing is to determine whether the patient has hyperpathia, pain that has an delayed onset, increases in intensity with repeated stimuli, and/or that continues (aftersensation) for some time (seconds, minutes) after discontinuation of the stimuli. Any 1 or more of these 3 phenomena indicates a hyperpathic response. The stimulus is applied repeatedly by gently touching the test area with the wooden end of a cotton swab stick (generally about 10 applications at 1 stroke/s). Alternately, the test area can be repeatedly contacted with a Semmes-Weinstein pressure esthesiometer.

Level C testing evaluates responses to noxious mechanical or thermal stimuli. The test is conducted similarly to level C for the patient with decreased altered sensation (described earlier). At the normal threshold and the increased threshold, the patient describes a sensation or displays a pain reaction out of proportion to the stimulus applied (ie, a pinprick seems like an electric shock or a searing, burning sensation, rather than simply a sharp pricking). Such description is termed hyperalgesia. Other than a 27-guage needle, alternative equipment for level C testing is as noted earlier.

In the patient who complains of unpleasant altered sensation and has documented abnormal painful responses to NST, local anesthetic blocks may be helpful in determining whether surgical intervention on the peripheral nerve suspected of being a causative factor in the patient's symptoms is indicated (Fig. 15). If a successful block of the nerve results in significant decrease or abolition of the patient's pain for the duration of the block, there is reason to believe that peripheral factors (ie, the injured peripheral nerve itself) are responsible for the pain and that the pain might be relieved or significantly lessened by exploration and repair of the nerve. If the pain is originating from an injury or prior operation in the neck and the patient has exhibited localized signs of sympathetic nervous system input (SMP/RSD, as discussed earlier), a stellate ganglion anesthetic block is administered. Relief of the pain after this block is diagnostic of RSD. Failure of the nerve blocks to produce significant pain relief indicates that the pain has a CNS component, there is development of collateral innervation, and/or it is related to psychological factors (so-called psychogenic pain) and that surgical intervention on the suspected peripheral nerve will not be successful in reducing or relieving it. In many cases, peripheral nerve surgery done after local anesthetic nerve blocks have failed to temporarily relieve pain results in an increase in the frequency, intensity, and/or duration of the patient's painful affliction.

Pictorial representation (mapping) of the results of NST in the patient's chart serves as an excellent method of preserving the responses to the various tests for comparison, if subsequent evaluations are indicated, and is easily done by making notes on standardized drawings on a printed examination form. Additional documentation in the form of patient photographs is often helpful for patients to monitor their progress/recovery following a nerve injury (Fig. 16).

Imaging

No evaluation of a peripheral nerve injury in the oral and maxillofacial region following an incident, dental procedure, or operation is complete without appropriate imaging of the structures in the vicinity of the injury. Depending on the indications and need for adequate diagnostic information, periapical or panoramic plain films, computed tomography, or magnetic resonance imaging may be

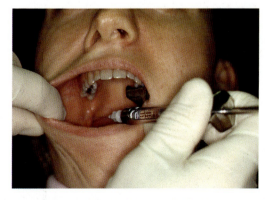

Fig. 15. The examiner is administering a local anesthetic block of the right IAN to assess its effect on the patient's neuropathic pain. The outcome of the nerve block may assist the clinician in decision making regarding nerve injury treatment, including possible microsurgical repair of the injured peripheral nerve (right IAN) suspected of being responsible for the patient's pain.

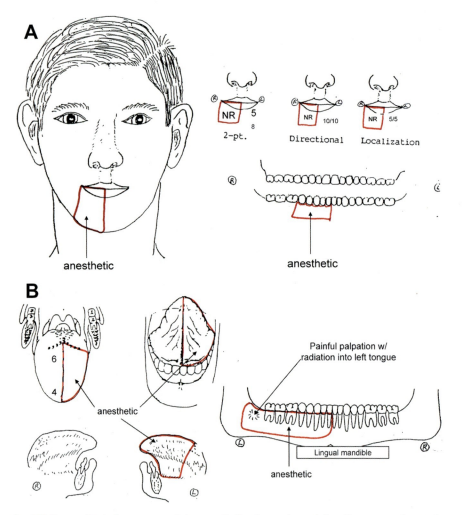

Fig. 16. After NST is completed, the responses of the area of altered sensation and the adjacent normal control areas are recorded in the patient's chart. Printed diagrams (mapping) are helpful in organizing and displaying the data for future reference. (*A*) Typical chart diagram showing a patient who has sustained a right IAN injury resulting in anesthesia (outlined in red) of the lower lip, chin, and mandibular labiobuccal mucosa. NR, no response or anesthetic. (*B*) Chart diagram of a patient who has sustained a left LN injury with anesthesia (outlined in red) of the anterior two-thirds of the left tongue, floor of mouth, and lingual gingiva. Note that there is a trigger area on lingual aspect of the left mandible with painful radiations into the left tongue. (*C*) (*Left*) Patient who presented 1 week following bilateral mandibular rami osteotomies and was found to have total anesthesia (outlined in red) of the distribution of the left IAN, as shown in this photograph. Seven weeks later the patient began to have symptoms and signs (to NST) of IAN recovery. (*Right*) At 6 months following her osteotomies, NST showed a much smaller area of altered sensation and normal responses to level B and level C testing. She continued to make progress without surgical intervention to recovery of satisfactory sensation by 1 year after nerve injury.

required. Examples of helpful information obtained from imaging studies during the evaluation of nerve-injured patients are shown in Fig. 17.

Diagnosis and classification

Correlation of all the information gathered during the evaluation will enable the clinician, either at the time of initial examination or after subsequent serial reevaluations, to make a diagnosis and classify the nerve injury.

The level of sensory impairment is identified at the appropriate stage along a spectrum from mild hypoesthesia to anesthesia. Painful injuries are designated as being caused by peripheral factors (and thus possibly amenable to surgical intervention), to sympathetic nervous system elements (RSD), or to CNS input.

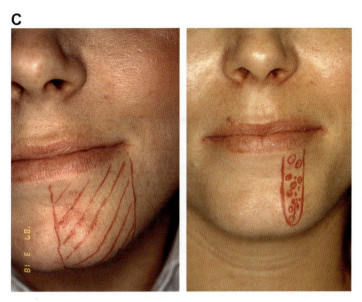

Fig. 16 (*continued*)

When peripheral nerve injuries are not directly observed at the time of their occurrence, subsequent serial examinations will provide the necessary information to classify the injury and provide guidance in the need for treatment. One classification of peripheral nerve injuries that the authors use in their practice, the Seddon classification, is shown in Table 2. In the Seddon classification, neurapraxia is a mild, temporary injury, likened to a concussion and often caused by

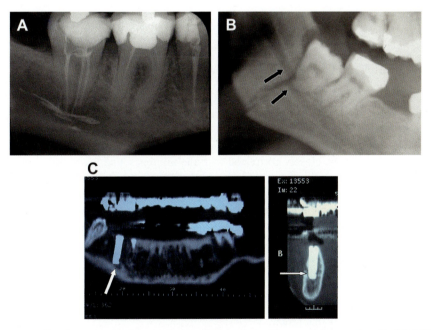

Fig. 17. Imaging studies done as part of the evaluation of the patient with nerve injury can provide helpful information regarding the location of the injury and assist in decision making regarding treatment. (*A*) Periapical film showing radiopaque material in the right IAC after endodontic treatment of the mandibular second molar. The axial spread of the material within the IAC usually indicates the extent of the IAN that has sustained a chemical burn. (*B*) Panoramic film of patient with mandibular angle fracture and significant offset of the proximal and distal inferior alveolar canal (*arrows*). If patient complains of sensory dysfunction in the ipsilateral lower lip and chin, a compression, crush, or laceration of the IAN at the fracture site should be strongly suspected and confirmed by NST. (*C*) Computed tomographic scan in the sagittal plane (*left*) shows possible contact of a dental implant with the mental foramen and/or inferior alveolar canal (*arrow*). In the coronal plane (*right*) there is definite encroachment of the implant on the MN (*arrow*).

Table 2
Seddon classification, adapted for peripheral trigeminal nerve injuries; comparison is made with the Sunderland classification (see text for discussion)

	Neurapraxia	Axonotmesis	Neurotmesis
Sunderland	I	II, III, IV	V
Nerve sheath	Intact	Intact	Interrupted
Axons	Intact	Some interrupted	All interrupted
Wallerian degeneration	None	Yes, some axons	Yes, all axons
Conduction failure	Transitory	Prolonged	Permanent
Spontaneous recovery	Complete	Partial	Poor to none
Time of recovery	Within 4 wk	Months	None, if not begun by 3 mo

compression or retraction of the nerve. Because spontaneous recovery usually occurs within 4 weeks, surgical intervention is not indicated. Axonotmesis is a more serious injury. Although the general structure of the nerve remains intact, there is loss of continuity of some axons, and they undergo Wallerian degeneration. There may be a partial failure of conduction or abnormality of speed of conduction. Initial symptoms and signs of nerve recovery do not begin until 1 to 3 months following injury. Eventual recovery is often less than normal (hypoesthesia), and, in the case of sensory nerve injury, development of dysesthesias is frequent. Microneurosurgical repair is helpful in improving decreased sensation or reducing pain in some patients. Neurotmesis is a complete transection or disruption of all layers of the nerve. There is Wallerian degeneration of most or all axons. There is a total conduction block that is permanent in most cases, unless there is surgical intervention. The Seddon classification is favored because it is based on the severity of nerve injury, time for recovery, and prognosis for recovery. It uses clinical information that is pertinent to those responsible for the care of such injuries, and it assists in making treatment decisions.

Readers are referred to Meyer and Ruggiero (2001) for a discussion of treatment based on the evaluation presented in this article.

Summary

This article presents a standardized method of clinical evaluation of the patient with a peripheral trigeminal nerve injury that provides both subjective and objective information. This evaluation scheme has been used by 1 author for more than 30 years (RAM) and by the other author (SCB) for 10 years. The information is easily obtained and recorded in the patient's record, and it can be used by any clinician who performs subsequent evaluations on the same patient. The NST methods have been used successfully by specialists in other surgical disciplines for many years, and the various test results have been found to be closely correlated with the injuries found when the responsible nerve was surgically explored.

Alternate testing methods or equipment are available that are used primarily in clinical and laboratory research rather than clinical practice. The reader who is interested in more information is encouraged to consult (Further Readings).

Acknowledgments

The authors wish to thank Courtney Pittman, CST, for her assistance in producing the clinical examination photographs for this article.

Further readings

Bagheri SC, Meyer RA, Ali Khan H, et al. Microsurgical repair of trigeminal nerve injuries from maxillofacial trauma. J Oral Maxillofac Surg 2009;67:1791.

Bagheri SC, Meyer RA, Ali Khan H, et al. Retrospective review of microsurgical repair of 222 lingual nerve injuries. J Oral Maxillofac Surg 2010;68:715.

Birch R, Bonney G, Wynn Parry CB. Surgical disorders of the peripheral nerves. Edinburgh (UK): Churchill-Livingstone; 1998.

Boyne PJ. Postexodontia osseous repair involving the mandibular canal. J Oral Maxillofac Surg 1982;40:69.

Campbell RL. The role of nerve blocks in the diagnosis of traumatic trigeminal neuralgia. Oral Maxillofac Surg Clin North Am 1992;4:369.

Cunningham LL, Tiner BD, Clark GM, et al. A comparison of questionnaire versus monofilament assessment of neurosensory deficit. J Oral Maxillofac Surg 1996;54:454.

Dyck PJ, Curtis DJ, Bushek W, et al. Description of "Minnesota Thermal Disks" and normal values of cutaneous thermal discrimination in man. Neurology 1974;24:325.

Essick GK. Comprehensive clinical evaluation of perioral sensory function. Oral Maxillofac Surg Clin North Am 1992;4:503.

Essick GK, Patel S, Trulsson M. Mechanosensory and thermosensory changes across the border of impaired sensitivity to pinprick after mandibular nerve injury. J Oral Maxillofac Surg 2002;60:1250.

Ghali GE, Epker BN. Clinical neurosensory testing: practical applications. J Oral Maxillofac Surg 1989;47:1074.

Gregg JM. Studies of traumatic neuralgia in the maxillofacial region: symptom complexes and response to microsurgery. J Oral Maxillofac Surg 1990;48:135.

Meyer RA. Discussion: studies of traumatic neuralgia in the maxillofacial region: symptom complexes and response to microsurgery. J Oral Maxillofac Surg 1990;48:141.

Meyer RA, Ruggiero SL. Guidelines for diagnosis and treatment of peripheral trigeminal nerve injuries. Oral Maxillofac Surg Clin North Am 2001;13:383.

Pogrel MA. Trigeminal evoked potentials and electrophysical assessment of the trigeminal nerve. Oral Maxillofac Surg Clin North Am 1992;4:535.

Posnick JC, Zimbler AG, Grossman JA. Normal cutaneous sensibility of the face. Plast Reconstr Surg 1990;86:429.

Robinson RC, Williams CW. Documentation method for inferior alveolar and lingual nerve paresthesias. Oral Surg Oral Med Oral Pathol 1986;62:128.

Seddon HJ. Nerve lesions complicating certain closed bone injuries. JAMA 1947;135:691.

Sunderland S. A classification of peripheral nerve injuries produced by loss of function. Brain 1951;74:491.

Vriens JP, van der Glas HW. Extension of normal values on sensory function for facial areas using clinical tests on touch and two-point discrimination. Int J Oral Maxillofac Surg 2009;38:1154.

Zuniga JR, Chen N, Phillips CL. Chemosensory and somatosensory regeneration after lingual nerve repair in humans. J Oral Maxillofac Surg 1997;55:2.

Zuniga JR, Meyer RA, Gregg JM, et al. The accuracy of clinical neurosensory testing for nerve injury diagnosis. J Oral Maxillofac Surg 1998;56:2.

Inferior Alveolar and Lingual Nerve Imaging

Michael Miloro, DMD, MD*, Antonia Kolokythas, DDS

Department of Oral and Maxillofacial Surgery, University of Illinois at Chicago, 801 South Paulina Street, MC 835, Chicago, Illinois 60612, USA

At present, there are no "purely" objective testing modalities available for evaluation of iatrogenic injury to the terminal branches of the trigeminal nerve, and this makes the clinical diagnosis and management of these conditions fairly complicated for the oral and maxillofacial surgeon. All available clinical neurosensory testing modalities require patient cooperation and are based on a patient response, thus introducing a subjective component to the "objective" process. Furthermore all testing is commonly performed at the post-injury stage, so no individual baseline testing results are available for comparison and true determination of the magnitude of the resultant damage. For objective testing, several imaging modalities are available and can assist in the preoperative risk assessment of the trigeminal nerve, as related the commonly performed procedures in the vicinity of the nerve, mostly third molar surgery. In addition, these studies may be applied for objective functional monitoring of either spontaneous or surgically assisted recovery of the inferior alveolar (IAN) and lingual (LN) branches of the third division of the trigeminal nerve. This article provides a review of all available imaging modalities and their clinical application relative to the preoperative nerve injury risk assessment, and postinjury and postsurgical repair recovery status of the IAN and LN.

General considerations

Because the LN and IAN are at risk for injury during a variety of common oral and maxillofacial surgical procedures, including third molar removal, interest in documenting the position of these specific nerves prior to surgery has been significant. Early attempts at documenting the position of the LN in the third molar region have included cadaveric dissections and clinical observations during third molar extraction surgery. These studies suffer from a variety of methodological problems, including the potential for iatrogenic displacement of the nerves during the surgical dissection (in both the cadaveric studies and the clinical trials) as well as from the cadaveric specimen fixation process. Despite these limitations, Kisselbach and Chamberlain reported the position of the LN in the third molar region in 34 cadaver specimens and 256 cases of third molar extraction. This study found that in 17.6% of cadaver specimens and in 4.6% of clinical cases, the LN was superior to the lingual crest, and in 62% of cases the LN was in direct contact with the lingual cortex. In another anatomic study, Pogrel and colleagues examined the LN position in the third molar region using reproducible landmarks in 20 cadavers (40 sides), and found the LN above the lingual crest in 15% of cases and a mean horizontal distance from the lingual crest of 3.45 mm. Both of these anatomic studies confirmed the relative vulnerable position of the LN during third molar surgery.

Objective, noninvasive, radiologic imaging modalities in the preoperative assessment of the patient at risk for nerve injury, as well as a method for monitoring following injury and postrepair phases of neurosensory recovery, are highly desirable. Radiologic assessment should be categorized with regard to the timing of the imaging period; that is, preinjury, postinjury, and postrepair phases. Preinjury assessment refers to the documentation of the in situ position of a nerve before any surgical

---

* Corresponding author.
E-mail address: mmiloro@uic.edu

intervention that may place that nerve at risk for iatrogenic injury (eg, third molar removal). Intraoperative monitoring of nerve function during a surgical procedure (eg, sagittal split mandibular osteotomy) that involves a specific nerve may also be used, most commonly with a functional assessment of nerve conduction and electrophysiological status, such as with somatosensory evoked potentials. Postinjury imaging may be divided into a primary phase (following nerve injury and allowing for spontaneous neurosensory recovery without microneurosurgical intervention) and a secondary phase (following surgical nerve exploration and microneurosurgical repair). Primary postinjury imaging may be clinically significant if it can correlate objective (radiologic) findings with subjective (clinical examination) findings, and thereby guide the need for microneurosurgical intervention and possibly aid in treatment planning (ie, the length of altered neural anatomy and the need for an interpositional nerve graft). In general, based on clinical neurosensory testing, an attempt is made to classify the injury according to one or more staging, or classification, schemes. The staging systems of Seddon and Sunderland are based on histologic assessment of nerve injury, and are intended to serve as prognostic indicators of the potential for spontaneous neurosensory recovery.

There have been several reports of intraoperative nerve monitoring specifically during LeFort osteotomy (V_2 division) and mandibular sagittal split osteotomy (V_3 division) procedures. These studies have used somatosensory evoked potentials to document the transient increased latency and decreased amplitude of signal activity that occurs during surgical manipulation of the nerve during the osteotomy procedures. Somatosensory evoked potentials can be used as a postinjury or postrepair test, to document the degree of neural injury and to monitor the progression of neurosensory recovery over time.

Preoperative radiologic risk assessment of the IAN and LN

Panoramic Radiography

The preoperative assessment of the position of the IAN during third molar consultation has been routinely performed with the use of a panoramic radiograph. Obviously the information gained from this study is extremely limited due to the 2-dimensional nature of the image, the variable magnification of the bony anatomy (for the IAN), and the complete inability to visualize the position of the lingual nerve. It should be kept in mind that this radiograph demonstrates the position of the inferior alveolar canal, and not the IAN, specifically. Valuable information can be obtained from the panoramic radiograph as a stand-alone imaging modality with regard to the relationship of the IAN in the vertical plane, but not in the horizontal dimension. The most useful aspect of the panoramic radiograph is in assessing increased potential for inferior alveolar nerve injury during third molar extraction based on the presence of several radiographic predictors (Fig. 1).

Other types of plain radiographs, such as periapical (Fig. 2) or anteroposterior films and lateral cephalograms, are not routinely used for accurate preoperative routine risk assessment for IAN injury. Superimposition and wide variations in magnification of the structures based on their location do not allow for reliable and reproducible information to be obtained with plain films. Furthermore, even if the IAN could be visualized in the third molar region, only a rough outline of tooth and root anatomy would be obtained, making these images of limited if any value for nerve injury appraisal.

Computed Tomography

The use of computed tomography (CT) in the assessment of nerve injuries is very limited, although it has been used more recently for assessment of the inferior alveolar canal with regard to the position of the third molar. An evaluation of bone window attenuation images may indicate violation of the cortical outline of the inferior alveolar canal, either from implant placement or following facial trauma (eg, posterior mandible fracture) (Fig. 3), but yields little information regarding the condition of the IAN itself or the neurovascular bundle. The use of soft tissue window CT images for the LN or IAN is compromised by very poor-detail resolution that precludes its routine application in neural assessment. Furthermore, dental artifacts often pose severe limitations in obtaining accurate information regarding the position of the LN to the lingual cortex of the mandible in critical areas, even in the soft tissue window views, and despite the current use of high-resolution image acquisition.

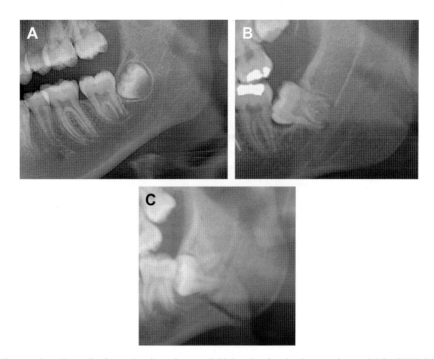

Fig. 1. (*A*) Panoramic radiograph of complete bony impacted third molar showing increased potential for IAN injury with loss of superior cortical outline of the inferior alveolar canal in the region of the third molar. (*B*) Panoramic radiograph of impacted third molar with radiographic predictors including loss of superior cortical outline of the inferior alveolar canal and darkening of the third molar roots. (*C*) Panoramic radiograph of left mandible fracture associated with an impacted third molar showing mild displacement and discontinuity of the inferior alveolar canal.

In 1998 CT cone beam (CBCT) technology, previously used only in angiographic imaging, was employed in the United States as a potential imaging modality for the maxillomandibular complex. The presurgical evaluation of impacted mandibular third molar relationship to the IAN has gained popularity over conventional CT scanning and plain panoramic radiographs among oral and maxillofacial surgeons. The need for accurate imaging with the lowest possible dose of radiation (ie, ALARA rule: As Low As Reasonably Achievable) seems to be satisfied acceptably with this technology. CBCT provides the desirable 3-dimensional representation of the anatomic location of interest, with minimal distortion compared with traditional plain films and by simpler acquisition compared with traditional CT systems. Similar to the panoramic radiograph, CBCT can be used for preoperative risk assessment in various dentoalveolar procedures such as third molar surgery or dental implants and preprosthetic surgery. A major limitation, of course, remains the inability to visualize

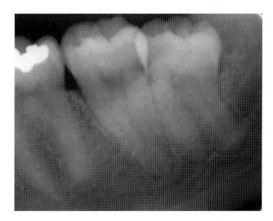

Fig. 2. Periapical radiograph showing proximity of third molar roots to the inferior alveolar canal, with root darkening.

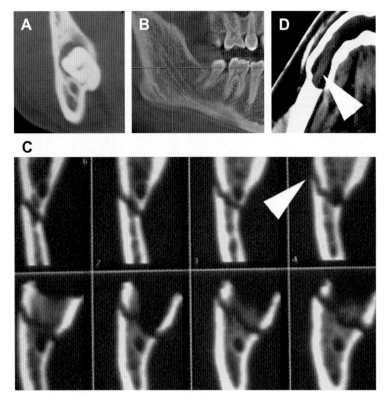

Fig. 3. (*A*) CT cone beam (CBCT) scan with coronal soft tissue window cuts showing impacted third molar and inferior alveolar canal, with the inability to discern any components of the inferior alveolar neurovascular bundle. (*B*) CBCT scan sagittal image with improved-detail resolution of the inferior alveolar canal position. (*C*) CT scan with coronal bony window cuts showing mandibular fracture involving the inferior alveolar canal (*arrowhead*). (*D*) CT scan with axial soft tissue window cuts in a patient with a cystic lesion of the mandible showing the inferior alveolar neurovascular bundle without significant detail (*arrowhead*).

the IAN itself (within the inferior alveolar canal), or the LN, because no accurate soft tissue information can be obtained with use of CBCT (Fig. 4).

High-Resolution Magnetic Resonance Imaging

Magnetic resonance imaging (MRI) is the method of choice for visualization of all cranial nerves (CN), and each nerve segment can be seen and examined in detail with specific MR sequences. Due to the complexity of the course and surrounding anatomic structures, detailed examination of the CNs

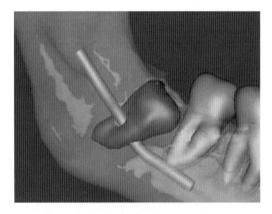

Fig. 4. Three-dimensional reformatted CBCT showing the course of the inferior alveolar canal between the impacted third molar roots.

is made possible only with careful planning and selection of the specific MRI technique. The imaging plane, coil selection, slice selection, in-plane resolution, and use of special techniques can be tailored based on the individual CN and the segment of interest so that the highest possible image quality may be obtained. The trigeminal nuclei (intra-axial), cisternal (preganglionic), and Merckel cave (intradural) segments contain both the motor and sensory components of the trigeminal nerve and can be visualized with high-resolution T1- or T2-weighted MR images. At the anterior aspect of the Gasserian ganglion, the sensory root divides into the ophthalmic, maxillary, and mandibular divisions, and each may be followed and examined separately based on their known course peripherally. The course of the LN and IAN branches of the mandibular division, after it exits from foramen ovale, can be followed with high-resolution, contrast-enhanced, T1-weighted (T1W), or T1W 3-dimensional, fast-filled echo (T1W 3D-FFE) sequences in the axial, coronal, and sagittal or parasagittal planes. Although detailed information can be obtained with the use MRI, routine presurgical evaluation of the route and integrity of the LN and IAN is not undertaken. Rather, the MRI is employed as the preferred imaging modality for examination of the status of the CNs, most commonly in the presence of a disease process or following brain injury.

Miloro and colleagues have used high-resolution MRI (HR-MRI) in an attempt to document the in situ position of the LN in the third molar region directly, without surgical manipulation or tissue distortion artifact as in the studies by Kisselbach and Pogrel. Ten patients (20 sides) without prior dental surgery were imaged using an HR-MRI sequence (PETRA-phase encoded time reduction acquisition) that enabled direct visualization of the LN (Fig. 5). This study documented that the lingual nerve position, while variable, was indeed vulnerable during third molar surgery; the LN was found to be superior to the lingual crest in 10% of cases, and in direct contact with the lingual plate in 25% of cases. Kress and colleagues have been able to image the IAN using T2-weighted MRI to visualize the IAN (Fig. 6).

Ultrasonography

Several reports have described the use of ultrasonography (US) and high-resolution ultrasound technology mainly for assessment of peripheral nerve lesions. This real-time advanced technology, with recently available high-resolution probes, can offer compound imaging without radiation and in a relatively inexpensive manner. Although US has not been employed or investigated as a potential preoperative risk assessment tool for the trigeminal nerve, it has been demonstrated to be valuable in identification and safe advancement of the needle in brachial plexus and sciatic nerve blocks. It would be reasonable, though, to anticipate limitations with the use of US in examination of the IAN in the third molar region, due to the presence of bone and teeth that might affect the echogenic signal. Visualization and documentation of the course and integrity of the LN, on the other hand, should be relatively easy, requiring only minimal training and familiarity of the operator with the regional oral anatomy.

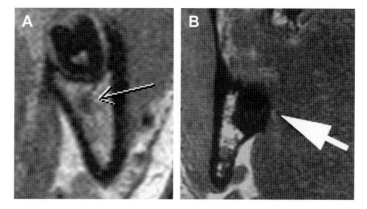

Fig. 5. (*A*) High-resolution MRI (HR-MRI) image in the third molar region showing minimal detail of the inferior alveolar neurovascular bundle (*arrow*). (*B*) HR-MRI image in the third molar region. Arrow indicates lingual nerve in direct contact with the lingual cortical plate.

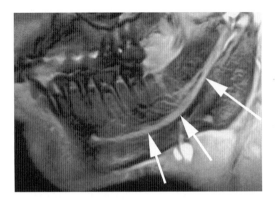

Fig. 6. Sagittal mandibular MRI image of a normal inferior alveolar nerve (*arrows*). (*Adapted from* Kress B, Gottschalk A, Stippich C, et al. MR imaging of traumatic lesions of the inferior alveolar nerve in patients with fractures of the mandible. AJNR Am J Neuroradiol 2003;24:1636; with permission.)

Postinjury radiographic assessment of the IAN and LN

The majority of current interest is in documenting the postinjury condition of the nerve by objective means, because the information gathered by clinical and radiologic examination could be useful in staging the degree of neural injury, determining the prognosis for recovery, and planning microneurosurgical intervention. With increased image resolution, the precise degree of architectural disruption of the nerve could be visualized and surgical intervention could be planned accordingly. In addition, this information could be used to document the exact location of the injury prior to surgical exploration for repair. For example, this documentation could help to avoid surgical nerve exploration in the third molar region if the injury occurred in the pterygomandibular space as a result of a mandibular block injection injury. Finally, radiologic techniques could be used to objectively monitor neurosensory progression, in conjunction with clinical examination, either after nerve injury or in the postrepair phases of neural recovery.

Panoramic Radiography

The postsurgery assessment of the nerve-injured patient usually includes a panoramic radiograph that may demonstrate a variety of clinically significant findings. The presence of a foreign body in the region of one or both nerves must be ruled out; these may include metallic foreign bodies from rotary instruments or amalgam particles from neighboring teeth, as well as retained tooth or root fragments following third molar surgery. Also, the presence of iatrogenic surgical disturbances of the nerves may be indicated by evidence of bone removal in proximity to the inferior alveolar neurovascular bundle or the lingual nerve (Fig. 7). However, a panoramic radiograph, or any other plain film, is rarely used to monitor progression following nerve injury or repair.

Computed Tomography

Postoperative investigation of the surgical site for examination of the integrity of the IAN canal or presence of foreign material, such as tooth or root fragments within the canal, could be superior and more reliable with CT or CBCT imaging than with use of traditional panoramic imaging. Direct investigation of the integrity of the LN cannot be reliably examined with either modality, because there is no bony conduit surrounding the nerve. Disruption of the lingual cortex of the mandible at the third molar region, which may be noted on a postoperative panoramic radiograph and which may imply iatrogenic injury in the region, can be reviewed in more detail with CT or CBCT. Direct comparisons of pre- and postoperative images can be made and be added to the information gathered from the clinical examination, and potentially assist in the decision-making process for surgery.

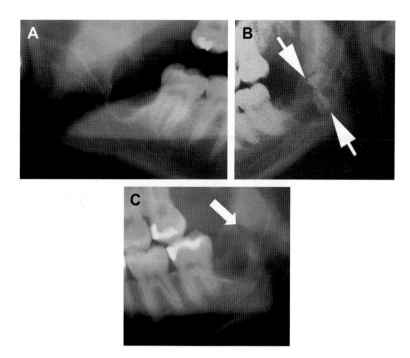

Fig. 7. (A) Panoramic radiograph post extraction, showing evidence the presence of radiographic predictors of potential IAN injury. (B) Panoramic radiograph showing retained root tips following third molar extraction (arrows) that may impede neural regeneration. (C) Panoramic radiograph showing evidence of bone removal distal to the third molar socket (arrow) in a patient with a left lingual nerve injury.

Magnetic Source Imaging

One of the few objective radiologic studies that are capable of documenting IAN injuries involves the use of magnetic source imaging (MSI), which combines magnetoencephalography (MEG) and HR-MRI. MEG technology uses magnetic fields to measure electrical brain activity and is influenced less by intervening soft tissues than electroencephalography (EEG), and therefore produces a more detailed image with higher resolution. Similar to somatosensory evoked potentials, a stimulus is applied peripherally (to the lower lip or tongue), and a signal is recorded centrally over the cerebral cortex; this enables measurement of signal latency and amplitude. The information obtained from MEG is combined with HR-MRI images to produce a structural and functional MSI of a particular region of the brain (Fig. 8). McDonald and colleagues employed MSI on 6 patients with unilateral IAN injury, and demonstrated that MSI technology may be able to differentiate various grades of neural injury. The findings on clinical examination and MSI imaging were correlated with surgical findings, and neural continuity defects were identified as radiographically different from intact

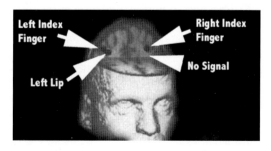

Fig. 8. Magnetic source image (MSI) in a patient with a right IAN injury showing lack of cortical signal (arrowhead). The right and left index fingers serve as controls. (Adapted from McDonald AR, Roberts TPL, Rowley HA, et al. Noninvasive somatosensory monitoring of the injured inferior alveolar nerve using magnetic source imaging. J Oral Maxillofac Surg 1996;54:1070; with permission.)

nerves. Despite some limitations of the study design (eg, small number, lack of blinded examiners and surgeons, and other study design flaws), there is potential for MSI to be applied in the postinjury and postrepair phases to monitor the progression of neurosensory recovery.

High-Resolution Magnetic Resonance Imaging

The application of HR-MRI to the assessment of the nerve following injury is in the early phases of clinical trials. The expectation is that with improved image resolution, a variety of anatomic changes in the nerve may be visualized. First, a change in nerve diameter may be visualized in cases of nerve injury with Wallerian degeneration of the nerve segment distal to the site of injury, with an acute or gradual decrease in nerve diameter. Second, an acute change in nerve position may be seen, for example where the lingual nerve is retracted into the region of the third molar socket with the formation of a lateral adhesive or exophytic neuromatous segment. Third, a change in nerve shape, for example, in a case of a fusiform neuroma-in-continuity where a change in shape of the nerve for a certain distance with return to normal shape distal to the neuroma, may be able to be visualized; thereby the length of nerve resection required can be planned, as well as the possible need for indirect nerve grafting using a sural nerve, or possibly a cadaveric nerve allograft.

The application of HR-MRI to postinjury neural assessment is currently hindered by a variety of factors. The degree of image resolution and magnification significantly limits precise anatomic examination of the individual neural elements. The ability to image the internal architecture of neural anatomy will require dramatic improvements in resolution over currently available techniques. Also, whereas the LN lies within soft tissue and its course is unaccompanied other than by the chorda tympani branch of the facial nerve, the IAN lies within a cortical bony conduit and is accompanied by an artery and a vein throughout its intrabony course. Preliminary studies with HR-MRI have allowed gross visualization of the LN because it is the sole structure in the area, but examination of the IAN has been complicated by the presence of the vessels, although attempts to attenuate the image signal may be able to overcome this problem, possibly with the use of magnetic resonance neurography (MRN). Depending on the plane of image section, HR-MRI may miss several anatomic indicators that a nerve injury has occurred. Individual transverse (or coronal, in the case of the LN in the third molar region) sections of the nerve may not visualize a short discontinuity or abrupt alteration in course of the nerve, depending on the distance between images. This problem may be avoided with the use of a sagittal, or longitudinal, image oriented along the course of the individual nerve. However, this is difficult because the position of the nerve varies normally in the uninjured patient, and may change significantly in the injured patient, thereby requiring either repositioning of the patient or redirection of the imaging plane.

The use of a noninvasive HR-MRI, with the lack of radiation exposure, for the nerve-injured patient would provide the advantage of correlating the results of clinical neurosensory testing and subjective patient evaluation, with an objective assessment of the anatomy of the injured nerve site. While it may seem that a frank transection injury (Sunderland Grade V) might be visualized easily with HR-MRI, the less severe injuries (Sunderland Grades III and IV) may be extremely difficult to discern and quantify radiographically. Future study designs with HR-MRI should include an experimental group of patients after nerve injury who undergo clinical neurosensory testing and HR-MRI, and then microneurosurgical nerve exploration and repair if indicated. This approach would allow correlation of postinjury radiologic results and findings at the time of nerve repair surgery to determine the ability of HR-MRI to accurately predict the actual degree of anatomic nerve injury. HR-MRI might also prove useful in monitoring the progression of anatomic neurosensory recovery (correlated with clinical signs and subjective symptoms) following nerve injury and/or microneurosurgical repair. Kress and colleagues have used MRI in cases of mandible fractures and following third molar removal to assess individual nerve fiber disruption in cases of mandible fracture, and changes in signal intensity following third molar extractions (Fig. 9).

Magnetic Resonance Neurography

Following the application of MRI technology to blood vessels, or magnetic resonance angiography (MRA), direct imaging of nerves with MRN was a logical technological progression. The MRN images are obtained using axial, coronal, and longitudinal T1 and T2 image acquisition with

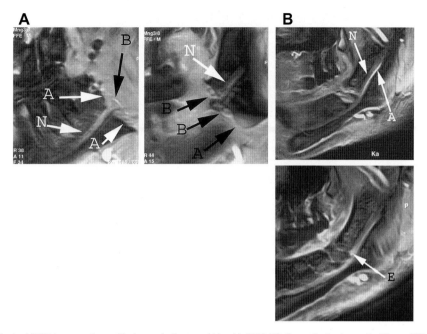

Fig. 9. (*A*) Sagittal MRI images of mandibular angle fracture (A), with IAN (N) discontinuity (note significant difference in the position of the IAN in each view), and possibly individual ruptured nerve fibers (B). (*B*) Sagittal T1 MRI images following third molar removal with intraventricular contrast injection to distinguish the inferior alveolar nerve (N) from the artery (A). There is evidence of signal increase in the IAN near the third molar extraction site (E). (*Adapted from* Kress B, Gottschalk A, Stippich C, et al. MR imaging of traumatic lesions of the inferior alveolar nerve in patients with fractures of the mandible. AJNR Am J Neuroradiol 2003;24:1636; and Kress B, Gottschalk A, Anders L, et al. High-resolution dental magnetic resonance imaging of inferior alveolar nerve responses to the extraction of third molars. Eur Radiol 2004;14:1419; with permission.)

customized phased array coils and imaging protocols. The application of MRN relies on its ability to distinguish nerves from surrounding structures such as blood vessels, lymph nodes, ligaments, adipose tissue, and ducts. This advantage would allow isolation of the inferior alveolar nerve from the neighboring artery and vein contained within the inferior alveolar bony canal. The MRN studies to date have documented the ability to distinguish intraneural from perineural masses, demonstrate nerve continuity versus discontinuity at the fascicular level, and localize extraneural nerve compression prior to nerve exploration. The majority of research has focused on larger, peripheral motor nerves including the brachial plexus, sciatic nerve, peroneal nerve, and femoral nerve. Filler and colleagues documented nerve compression and signal hyperintensity of an inferior alveolar nerve in a patient with a lymphoma of the pterygomandibular space (Fig. 10). MRN has been able to document an increased diameter of injured nerves as well as increased signal intensity, and longitudinal variations associated with nerve injury and recovery. There does not seem to be any correlation between the amount of hyperintensity and the degree of neural injury, and its significance has not yet been clearly defined. The finding of signal hyperintensity has been demonstrated for a transient period following neural anastomosis, as well as distal to a nerve graft site. The remarkable ability of MRN to depict fascicular architecture is based on the difference in fluid composition of the neural elements. The fascicles contain a preponderance of endoneurial fluid and axoplasmic water, while the interfascicular space is largely composed on fibrofatty connective tissue. In a sense, these images may be able to define radiographically the histologic characteristics of different grades of nerve injuries set forth by Seddon and Sunderland. Similarly, sequential images could be used to monitor nerve recovery at the fascicular level. One of the most advantageous characteristics of MRN images is the ability to image the nerve in a longitudinal plane. In a technique similar to that of an MRA used to image the anatomy of an abdominal aortic aneurysm, these MRN images can easily be assessed for variations in nerve anatomy, diameter, location, discontinuity, and signal intensity, which may indicate areas of nerve injury and thereby guide surgical intervention as well as monitor neurosensory recovery.

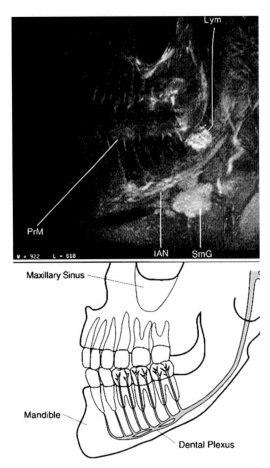

Fig. 10. Magnetic resonance neurogram showing increased signal in the pterygomandibular space from a lymphoma (*arrow*), and delineation of the inferior alveolar nerve (IAN). SmG, submandibular gland; PrM, premolar. (*Adapted from* Filler AG, Kliot M, Hayes CE, et al. Application of magnetic resonance neurography in the evaluation of patients with peripheral nerve pathology. J Neurosurg 1996;85:306; with permission.)

Ultrasonography

Recently some promising findings were reported with the use of US for visualization of the lingual trauma in the pig cadaver head. In the study by Olsen and colleagues, the iatrogenic injuries created were successfully categorized in 17 out of 27 attempts once the examiners became familiar with visualization of the LN (Fig. 11). The major remaining limiting factor in the use of US for such application is the lack of training and familiarity with the ultrasound technology and imaging among surgeons. The possibility of incorporating US for investigation of the integrity of LN postoperatively along with clinical evaluation seems promising. The potential for ultrasound examination in several subsequent visits in a noninvasive manner, without the need for radiation, additional cost, or discomfort, with the ability to document findings of every examination for comparison and evaluation of progression, make this modality reasonably valuable.

Postinjury functional assessment of the IAN and LN

Among the imaging modalities discussed thus far, it should be evident that the only ones that could potentially contribute to the functional assessment of the postrepair nerve are MRI-HR, functional MRI/MRN, and US technology. Success or failure of grafting or direct anastomosis after nerve repair can be assessed only after several months have elapsed and are based on neurosensory examination.

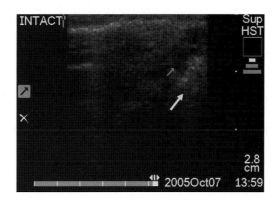

Fig. 11. Ultrasonography image of lingual nerve (*upper arrow*) above the lingual crest of the mandible (*lower arrow*). (*Adapted from* Olsen J, Papadaki M, Troulis, M, et al. Using ultrasound to visualize the lingual nerve. J Oral Maxillofac Surg 2007;65 (11):2299; with permission.)

The use of MRN has been proved valuable to evaluate the repair site for neuroma formation or problems with the sutures when there is no recovery, and to direct the need for early intervention. With the current advances in MRN, the few limitations posed by the presence of hematoma in the early phases of repair initially discussed in the literature are no longer an issue. Finally, nerve continuity after direct repair or interpositional grafting can be examined with US, but more details can be obtained with MRN. Once again a major limitation with the use of US is the lack of training among surgeons in familiarity with the acquired images for appropriate interpretation.

The current advances in MRI technology with high-resolution, functional, or metabolic-based images (BOLD: Blood Oxygenation Level Dependent) certainly allow for detailed examination of the neural structures, pathology, and injury. Perhaps the main potential limitations in routine use of these advanced applications for investigation of IAN and LN injuries and recovery would be the cost associated with the studies, and the lack of familiarity of the neuroradiologists and surgeons regarding their endless possibilities.

Although current ability to image the IAN and LN with precision, detail, and accuracy is limited, with the rapid development of technological advancements and improvements in imaging modalities, 3-dimensional imaging capabilities that will effectively image both the IAN and LN will certainly come about. Also, functional neural and brain imaging will allow correlation of the clinical examination with direct anatomic and physiologic functional parameters.

Further readings

Dailey A, Tsuruda JS, Filler AG, et al. Magnetic resonance neurography of peripheral nerve degeneration and regeneration. Lancet 1997;350:1221–2.

Dailey AT, Tsuruda JS, Goodkin R, et al. Magnetic resonance neurography for cervical radiculopathy: a preliminary report. Neurosurgery 1996;38:488–92.

Filler AG, Howe FA, Hayes CE, et al. Magnetic resonance neurography. Lancet 1993;341:659–61.

Filler AG, Kliot M, Hayes CE, et al. Application of magnetic resonance neurography in the evaluation of patients with peripheral nerve pathology. J Neurosurg 1996;85:299–309.

Filler AG, Maravilla KR, Tsuruda JS. MR neurography and muscle MR imaging for image diagnosis of disorders affecting the peripheral nerves and musculature. Neurol Clin 2004;22(3):643–82, vi–vii.

Garbedian J. The relationship of the lingual nerve to the 3rd molar region: a three dimensional analysis. In: Graduate Department of Dentistry. Toronto: University of Toronto; 2009. p. 95.

George JS, Aine CJ, Mosher JC. Mapping function in the human brain with magnetoencephalography, anatomical magnetic resonance imaging, and functional magnetic resonance imaging. J Clin Neurophysiol 1995;12:406.

Ghaeminia H, Meijer GJ, Soehardi A, et al. Position of the impacted third molar in relation to the mandibular canal. Diagnostic accuracy of cone beam computed tomography compared with panoramic radiography. Int J Oral Maxillofac Surg 2009; 38(9):964–71.

Graif M, Seton A, Nerubai J, et al. Sciatic nerve: sonographic evaluation and anatomic-pathologic considerations. Radiology 1991;181:405–8.

Grant GA, Britz GW, Goodkin R, et al. The utility of magnetic resonance imaging in evaluating peripheral nerve disorders. Muscle Nerve 2002;25:314–31.

Hayes CE, Tsuruda JS, Mathis CM, et al. Brachial plexus: MR imaging with a dedicated phased array surface coil. Radiology 1997;203:286–9.

Howe FA, Filler AG, Bell BA, et al. Magnetic resonance neurography. Magn Reson Med 1992;28:328–38.

Howe FA, Saunders D, Filler AG, et al. Magnetic resonance neurography of the median nerve. Br J Radiol 1994;67:1169–72.

Jaaskelainen SK, Teerijoki-Oksa T, Forssell K, et al. Intraoperative monitoring of the inferior alveolar nerve during mandibular sagittal-split osteotomy. Muscle Nerve 2000;23:368–75.

Kiesselbach JE, Chamberlain JG. Clinical and anatomic observations on the relationship of the lingual nerve to the mandibular third molar region. J Oral Maxillofac Surg 1984;42:565–7.

Kress B, Gottschalk A, Anders L, et al. High-resolution dental magnetic resonance imaging of inferior alveolar nerve responses to the extraction of third molars. Eur Radiol 2004;14:1416–20.

Kress B, Gottschalk A, Stippich C, et al. MR imaging of traumatic lesions of the inferior alveolar nerve in patients with fractures of the mandible. AJNR Am J Neuroradiol 2003;24:1635–8.

Kuntz C, Blake L, Britz G, et al. Magnetic resonance neurography of peripheral nerve lesions in the lower extremity. Neurosurgery 1996;39:750–7.

Maloney SR, Bell WL, Shoaf SC, et al. Measurement of lingual and palatine somatosensory evoked potentials. Clin Neurophysiol 2000;111:291–6.

McDonald AR, Roberts TPL, Rowley HA, et al. Noninvasive somatosensory monitoring of the injured inferior alveolar nerve using magnetic source imaging. J Oral Maxillofac Surg 1996;54:1068–72.

Miloro M, Halkias LE, Chakeres DW, et al. Assessment of the lingual nerve in the third molar region using magnetic resonance imaging. J Oral Maxillofac Surg 1997;55:134–7.

Olsen J, Papadaki M, Troulis M, et al. Using ultrasound to visualize the lingual nerve. J Oral Maxillofac Surg 2007;65(11): 2295–300.

Pogrel MA, Renaut A, Schmidt B, et al. The relationship of the lingual nerve to the mandibular third molar region: an anatomic study. J Oral Maxillofac Surg 1995;53:1178–81.

Rood JP, Shehab AA. The radiological prediction of inferior alveolar nerve injury during third molar surgery. Br J Oral Maxillofac Surg 1990;28:20.

Seddon JJ. Three types of nerve injury. Brain 1943;66:237.

Slimp JC. Intraoperative monitoring of nerve repairs. Hand Clin 2000;16:25–36.

Sunderland S. A classification of peripheral nerve injuries produced by loss of function. Brain 1951;74:491.

Tanrikulu L, Hastreiter P, Richter P, et al. Virtual neuroendoscopy: MRI-based three-dimensional visualization of the cranial nerves in the posterior cranial fossa. Br J Neurosurg 2008;22(2):207–12.

Zuniga JR, Meyer RA, Gregg JM, et al. The accuracy of clinical neurosensory testing for nerve injury diagnosis. J Oral Maxillofac Surg 1998;56:2–8.

Management of Mandibular Nerve Injuries from Dental Implants

Shahrokh C. Bagheri, DMD, MD[a,b,c,d], Roger A. Meyer, DDS, MS, MD[e,*]

[a]Private Practice, Georgia Oral and Facial Surgery, 1880 West Oak Parkway, Suite 215, Marietta, GA 30062, USA
[b]Division of Oral & Maxillofacial Surgery, Department of Surgery, Northside Hospital, 1000 Johnson Ferry Road, Atlanta, GA 30342, USA
[c]Department of Surgery, School of Medicine, Emory University, 1365 Clifton Road NE, Atlanta, GA 30322, USA
[d]Department of Oral & Maxillofacial Surgery, School of Dentistry, Medical College of Georgia, 1120 15th Street, Augusta, GA 30912, USA
[e]Maxillofacial Consultations Ltd, 1021 Holt's Ferry, Greensboro, GA 30642, USA

Dental implant surgery has become the standard of care for reconstruction of simple and complex edentulous areas of the maxilla and mandible. The risks of injury to the branches of the mandibular division (MdN) of the trigeminal nerve (inferior alveolar nerve [IAN], lingual nerve [LN], and mental nerve [MN]) are known complications of implant restoration of the posterior mandible. The use of advanced imaging modalities such as cone beam computed tomography (CT) scans and high-definition panoramic radiographs can assist in localization of the inferior alveolar canal (IAC). However, despite correct planning, the possibility of injury to the MdN is not entirely eliminated. Sensory dysfunction, especially if persistent or painful, can be distressing to both the patient and the clinician. Altered sensation after implant surgery continues to bear medicolegal implications that further warrant the implantologist's attention. In the treatment of nerve injuries associated with dental implant surgery it is most important that there be prompt recognition and acknowledgment of the patient's sensory complaints and timely decisions regarding management to maximize the recovery of nerve function. The clinician is faced with 2 problems: (1) treatment of the neurosensory disturbance (NSD) of the affected region, and (2) how best to proceed with dental restoration of the affected area. Such patients are frequently distressed and disappointed in their treatment outcome. Their concerns are best addressed by a continuing supportive relationship with, and appropriate recommendations for further treatment from, their implantologist.

This article presents the causes and management of injuries to the MdN of the trigeminal nerve from dental implant surgery.

Causes and pathogenesis

The 4 most frequent causes of injury to the MdN related to dental implant surgery are errors in evaluation and planning, the injection of local anesthetic for the implant procedure, the bone preparation (drilling), and placement of the implant. Other reasons for nerve injury are also discussed.

Errors in Radiographic Planning

The panoramic radiograph is useful as the primary imaging study to assess the vertical distance from the crest of the mandibular alveolar ridge to the superior aspect of the IAC. The panoramic machine should be calibrated for distortion or magnification to allow accurate determination of

* Corresponding author.
E-mail address: rameyer@aol.com

dimensions from panoramic films. If the panoramic film shows inadequate distance from the alveolar crest to the IAC to support an implant cylinder, the mediolateral position of the IAC needs to be determined to decide whether an implant can be placed without repositioning of the IAN or MN (see later discussion). In such patients, a CT scan is a necessary part of the evaluation.

Regardless of the radiographic modality (CT or panoramic radiograph) used for implant planning, errors in interpretation and application of the radiograph can lead to unplanned implant positioning. The CT scans have improved resolution and allow visualization of the nerve in 3 dimensions. However, errors of software planning can be translated into the surgical procedure. Attention should be given to the accuracy of the surgical guides and their seating onto the alveolar ridge. Placement of the surgical guide on a totally edentulous mandible will have a significant inherent margin of error related to the soft tissue despite correct planning. It is important to allow an additional reasonable distance (ie, 2–3 mm) from the nerve during the CT planning to accommodate this margin of error. Although the use of flap-less surgery (Fig. 1) for implant placement using navigation guides is becoming popular, the surgeon should not hesitate to raise a mucoperiosteal flap to better visualize and confirm anatomic landmarks as needed.

Injection of Local Anesthetic

The IAN or LN can be injured secondary to the injection of a local anesthetic into the pterygomandibular space or the MN when injecting in the area of the mental foramen. Although the exact pathophysiology of this injury remains unknown, there are 3 possible causes: (1) direct intraneural injection with mechanical injury to the nerve (ie, severance of axons, partial or total, scar tissue or neuroma formation, Wallerian degeneration, and so forth), (2) interruption of vessels of the mesoneurium with peri- and intraneural hemorrhage and secondary scar formation, and (3) chemical toxicity of the anesthetic solution from a contaminant (sterilizing solution) in a leaky carpule. Regardless of its cause, it is recommended that aspiration be done before all local anesthetic injections. If there is a bloody aspirate or the patient complains of a paresthesia (typically, an electric shock-like sensation), the needle is withdrawn a few millimeters and aspiration is repeated. If there is now no bloody aspirate, it can be assumed that the needle tip is no longer in contact with a blood vessel or nerve, and the injection is completed. A note of such an occurrence should be routinely entered in the patient's chart. This technique may prevent direct injection into a vascular space, but does not necessarily prevent deposition of the anesthetic within the epineurium (the diameter of the IAN is 4–5 times greater than the associated inferior alveolar artery or vein). Nerve injury secondary to local anesthetic injection, although uncommon, has a reported incidence of 1:26,762 to 1:160,571. It can be difficult to differentiate from injury related to the placement of the dental implants, especially if the patient was under sedation or general anesthesia and, therefore, unable to report a paresthesia at the time of the injection(s). Without obvious clinical or radiographic signs of injury to the nerve, the possibility of needle injection injury cannot be eliminated. Unfortunately, a very small percentage of patients who have suffered an injection-related injury can be misdiagnosed with injury related to the dental implant surgery, and subsequently undergo diagnostic or exploratory surgical procedures that reveal no visible nerve injury at the implant location.

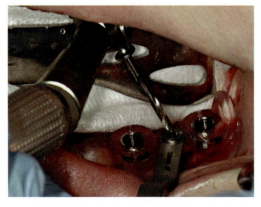

Fig. 1. Flap-less surgery for implant placement using navigation guides. Both the depth and the position of the osteotomy are determined by the guide.

Bone Preparation

Injury to the IAN as a consequence of bone preparation or implant placement can be caused by errors in radiographic planning, drilling, or direct contact of the implant with the nerve.

Drill injuries to the IAN can be difficult to diagnose. Despite correct position of the implant vis-à-vis the IAC on the postoperative radiograph appearance of the implant, osseous preparation with the drill may have been performed beyond the planned implant depth causing injury to the nerve (Fig. 2). This error can be prevented by correct radiographic measurement of the distance from the alveolar ridge crest to the superior aspect of the IAC, the use of drilling equipment with predetermined depth stops, and careful technique to prevent drilling beyond the planned depth. Irrigation with adequate coolant to dispel heat generated by bone drilling may also prevent a thermal injury in the absence of direct contact with the nerve. Frequent intraoperative reverification of the drill dimensions (diameter and length) is also helpful.

Implant Placement (Direct Implant Injury)

In addition to injury caused by drilling, the extent of injury of the IAN caused by the implant itself is related to the degree of encroachment of the implant into the IAC or its direct contact with the IAN (Fig. 3). Nerve injury caused by implant placement may occur, despite correct osseous preparation, when the implant is inserted beyond the vertical confines of the prepared bone, compressing or breaching the superior wall of the IAC and forcing bone into the canal (Fig. 4A). Alternately, extension of drilling into the IAC may facilitate over insertion of the implant cylinder beyond its intended depth and into the IAC, making direct contact with the IAN (see Fig. 4B, C). Delayed osseous healing and remodeling from localized injury can cause excess bone formation and compromise of the IAC cross-sectional diameter (see Fig. 4D).

Other Causes of Injury

The MN lies in the mandibular buccal soft tissue and is at risk of injury during incisions. Recognition of the changing anatomy of the edentulous mandible is particularly helpful in minimizing risk of injury to the MN. As the patient ages, the alveolar bone in an edentulous area resorbs, and the position of the mental foramen becomes closer to the crest of the alveolar ridge (Fig. 5A). In some patients there is actual dehiscence of the IAC, and the IAN and the MN come to lie on the alveolar ridge crest (see Fig. 5B). Placement of an incision must, therefore, take these anatomic changes into consideration. During the retraction of a mucoperiosteal flap it is possible to exert continuous undue pressure on the underlying MN. Gentle soft tissue retraction with frequent brief relaxation of retraction pressure is suggested (see Fig. 5C).

Less common causes of nerve injury are related to placement of bone grafts (autologous, allogenic, xenogenic) during simultaneous implant placement. In cases of complex implant reconstruction, the bone

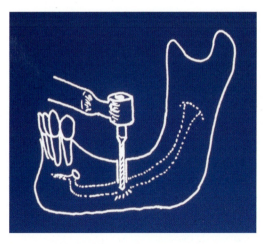

Fig. 2. Direct injury to the IAN by drilling beyond the planned osteotomy.

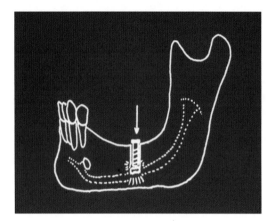

Fig. 3. Placement of the implant into the IAN (*arrow*).

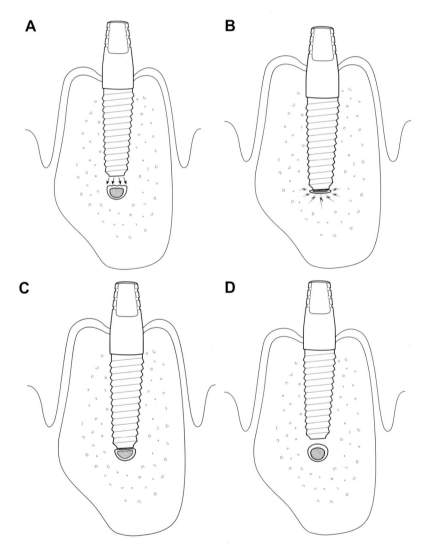

Fig. 4. (*A*) Collapse of the superior aspect of the IAC as a result of implant placement beyond the planned osteotomy causing injury to the nerve (compartment syndrome). (*B*) Direct injury. (*C*) Direct injury to the cortical rim of the IAC with deformation of the neurovascular bundle. (*D*) Remodeling of the IAC cortical rim causing narrowing of canal.

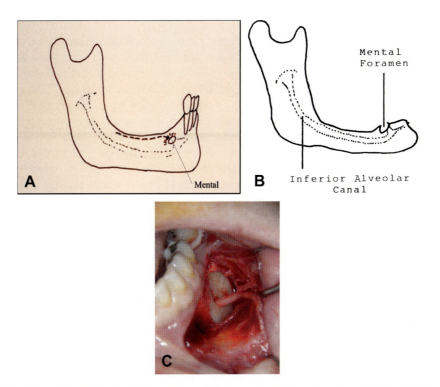

Fig. 5. (A) Superior position of the mental foramen caused by resorption of the alveolar bone in the partially edentulous mandible. (B) Dehiscence of the IAC, and the IAN and the MN come to lie on the alveolar ridge crest. (C) Exposure of the MN with gentle traction and frequent relaxation minimizes the chance of nerve injury.

graft material may be placed into the donor site with excessive force, thus severely compressing or even crushing the IAN. The authors have encountered several cases of particulate bone graft material within the IAC that caused significant nerve compression, and other cases of severe scarring, similar in clinical appearance to a chemical burn, when calcium hydroxyapatite came in direct contact with the nerve.

Evaluation of nerve injuries

Neurosensory disturbances are evaluated and documented in a standard fashion using the Medical Research Council Scale (MRCS) guidelines, as modified for the oral and maxillofacial regions, regardless of the cause of the sensory nerve injury. The evaluation of nerve injuries is discussed in a separate article by Meyer and Bagheri elsewhere in this issue.

Treatment

Timely repair of peripheral nerve injuries has always been the sine qua non for successful recovery of nerve function, especially since Seddon's extensive experience with treatment of missile injuries to extremities during and after World War II. His comment, "If a purely expectant policy is pursued, the most favorable time for operative intervention will always be missed..." is as pertinent today as it was more than 60 years ago. As in all other causes of nerve injury, treatment of the patient with a dental implant-associated nerve injury is dependent on the correct diagnosis of the injury and its timely management.

The perioperative administration of supportive medications has been advocated for patients undergoing procedures such as dental implants, mandibular osteotomies, and removal of lower third molars, which are associated with a risk of nerve injury. There is conflict in the literature between those who recommend beginning corticosteroids preoperatively and others who advise waiting postoperatively for several days before initiating administration. Many surgeons routinely give a single preoperative intravenous dose of a steroid (dexamethasone or hydrocortisone). Whether or not it is beneficial to initiate corticosteroid or antiinflammatory medications after a nerve injury has occurred is questionable. Previous studies have documented the lack of benefit of corticosteroids administered to reduce cerebral edema in patients who have sustained head injuries. That the IAN, in a similar closed box situation, confined within the IAC, could benefit from retroactively administered corticosteroid seems unlikely.

Our algorithm for the management of nerve injuries from dental implant surgery is shown in Fig. 6. The patient who complains of decreased or painful sensation following placement of dental implants should be requested to return to the office for evaluation. In some patients a nerve injury might have been suspected, if the patient complained of paresthesia during local anesthetic injection or during the bone drilling preparation for implant placement. In most cases, however, the patient is under intravenous sedation, and there is no indication during the procedure of a nerve injury. It is recommended that the patient be seen as soon as is convenient, preferably within 24 hours or the same day, if painful sensation is the chief complaint, so that adequate pain control can be established and rapport with the patient maintained. The exact nature of the patient's complaints should be ascertained (see article on evaluation by Meyer and Bagheri elsewhere in this issue). A general oral examination is performed to assess the healing status of the surgical site. Neurosensory testing (NST) is done to establish an objective baseline determination of the level of sensory dysfunction for further follow-up, as indicated.

A panoramic radiograph is obtained to determine the position of the implant(s) in relation to the IAN. If there is no close relationship of the implant and the IAC on the panoramic film, no repositioning or removal of the implant is indicated and should not be done. The patient is followed expectantly with frequent repeat NST to assess progress of recovery of sensation, if any. Those patients who go on to acceptable (to the patient) spontaneous recovery require no further active treatment. Patients who fail to regain acceptable sensory function within 3 (anesthesia) or 4 (hypoesthesia with or without pain) months are referred to a microsurgeon for possible nerve exploration and repair. If there is superimposition of the implant over the IAC on the panoramic film, a CT scan is done to determine whether this represents an encroachment on the IAN or IAC or simply a two-dimensional radiographic overlap that cannot be distinguished on the panoramic radiograph. If the CT demonstrates that the implant is not in contact with the IAC, the implant can be maintained and the patient is followed expectantly with serial NST to determine if spontaneous recovery occurs (see earlier discussion) (Fig. 7).

On the contrary, if the implant is in direct contact with the IAC, then the implant should be repositioned immediately (before osseointegration) to create at least 2-mm separation from the canal. This may allow the patient to maintain the implant despite the outcome of nerve injury. If the implant

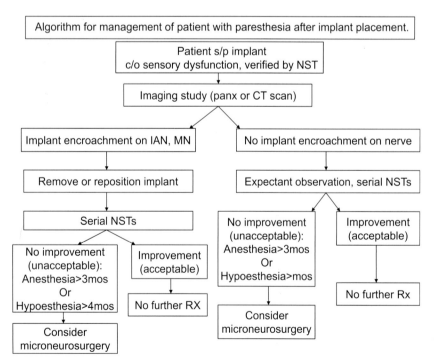

Fig. 6. Algorithm for the management of nerve injuries from dental implant surgery. NST, neurosensory testing; Panx, panoramic radiograph; Rx, treatment.

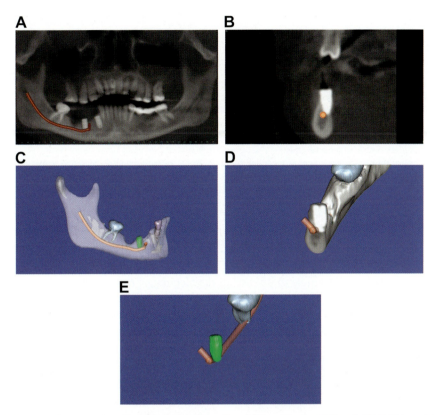

Fig. 7. (A) CT-generated panoramic radiograph demonstrating the position of implant #29 to the IAC. This patient presented with severe dysesthesia of the IAN. (B) Cross-sectional view (coronal) of the same patient demonstrating impingement of the implant to the IAN. (C) Three-dimensional reconstruction with transparency of the osseous structures showing the IAC and the implant. (D) Three-dimensional reconstruction in a cross section. (E) Three-dimensional reconstruction in cross section with removal of the osseous structures.

cannot be repositioned without compromising its stability, then it should be removed. The patient should be reevaluated with NST within 1 week. If there are signs of neurosensory recovery, no further treatment may be necessary, except for interval NST to document progress to satisfactory recovery (useful sensory function or better). The implant can be restored if it has adequate stability and meets prosthodontic criteria for restoration.

If, on removal or repositioning of the implant, the patient does not show acceptable signs of recovery within 3 (anesthesia) or 4 (hypoesthesia/pain) months by serial NST, microsurgical consultation is indicated. Because the IAN lies within a bony canal, spontaneous recovery might occur as a result of guided regeneration of the nerve provided by the confines of the canal. In such case, recovery of sensory function should begin (onset of symptoms, responses to NST) within 3 months after nerve injury. Microsurgical consultation can be considered earlier if there is a diagnosis of nerve transection (ie, by direct visualization at the time of surgery). The so-called 12-week rule for the anesthetic patient has subsequently come to be recognized by many surgeons who care for nerve injuries as the standard for timely decision making for the nerve injury patient who has an unacceptable persistent total loss of sensory function. The patient who still has partial but unacceptable recovery of sensation at 3 months after nerve injury can be followed at regular (1 month) intervals as long as there is progressive improvement in subjective symptoms and NST at each visit. Once improvement ceases, it will not resume at some indeterminate time in the future, and a treatment decision is made at that time, depending on the level of the sensory deficit to NST, the patient's subjective assessment and any associated functional impairment.

Surgical procedures for IAN injuries from dental implants

A list of microneurosurgical procedures that can provide surgical management of IAN injuries from dental implants is given in Table 1. Fig. 8A–J shows various microsurgical operations. Although

Table 1
Representative list of microneurosurgical procedures

Nerve operation	
External decompression	Removal of surrounding bony, soft tissue structures and/or foreign material around the nerve
Internal neurolysis	Opening of the epineurium to inspect and decompress the nerve fascicles
Excision of neuroma	Removal of a neuroma associated with a nerve
Neurorrhaphy	Microsurgical anastamosis of a transected nerve
Nerve graft	Placement of a nerve graft (allogenic or autogenous) for nerve reconstruction
Nerve sharing	Microsurgical anastamosis of a distal nerve to a different proximal nerve via an interposed nerve graft
Guided nerve regeneration	Placement of a conduit to guide axonal sprouting and regeneration across a nerve gap from proximal to distal portions of a nerve
Neurectomy	Microsurgical transection and removal of a segment of a peripheral nerve
Nerve capping	Covering of the proximal stump of a transected nerve with its epineurium to prevent neuroma formation
Nerve redirection	Redirection of a nerve's sensory innervation to a different anatomic location (usually adjacent muscle); usually done to prevent or minimize deafferentation

it is beyond the scope of this article to discuss all the techniques listed in Table 1, in our review of 186 IAN injuries (pending publication), the most commonly performed operation was autogenous (sural or great auricular) nerve grafts (n = 71, 38.2%) for reconstruction of nerve severance, followed by internal neurolysis (n = 60, 32.3%) when the nerve was not discontinuous.

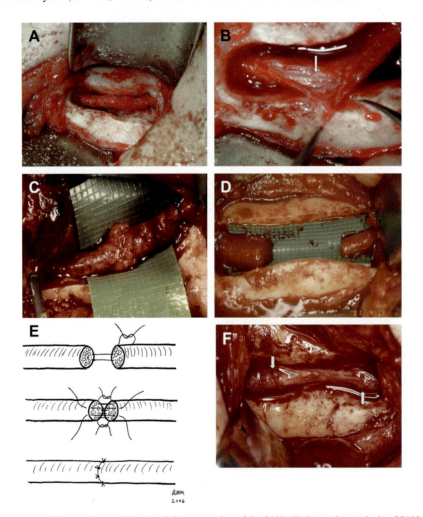

Fig. 8. Microneurosurgical procedures: (*A*) external decompression of the IAN; (*B*) internal neurolysis of IAN (*arrow*); (*C*) neuroma in continuity of the IAN; (*D*) IAN after excision of a neuroma in continuity; (*E*) direct neurorrhaphy; (*F*) sural nerve graft for the IAN reconstruction (*arrow*); (*G*) decellularized human nerve graft (Axogen, Alachua, FL, USA) for IAN reconstruction; (*H*) guided tissue regeneration; (*I*) neurectomy and nerve capping; (*J*) nerve redirection.

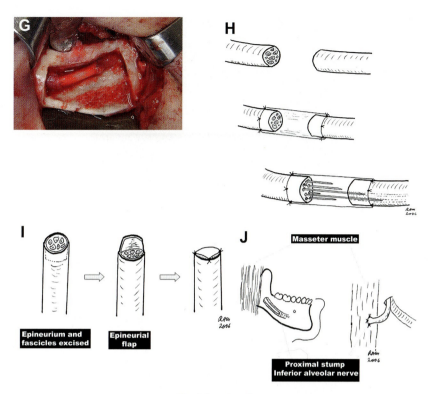

Fig. 8 (*continued*)

Nerve Exploration

High-resolution CT imaging can provide extensive detail of the bony anatomy, including the IAC. Magnetic resonance imaging (MRI) may be able to provide adequate visualization of the LN or MN. However, the ultimate view of the injured nerve requires visualization provided by surgical exploration. Exploration of the IAN will reveal any gross anatomic abnormalities, presence of bony fragments or foreign bodies (graft material) that may be impinging on the nerve, any contact of the nerve with the implant (Fig. 9) or the formation of scar tissue associated with the nerve (Fig. 10).

Removal of Implant

The technique of implant removal depends on whether the implant has osseointegrated or not. If the implant is fully osseointegrated, it is best removed using a trephine burr that cuts circumferentially around the implant allowing removal with minimal bone sacrifice. A recently placed implant that has not osseointegrated can be removed using a torque wrench or drill. Appropriate bone preservation techniques should be used for possible future implant replacement. However, care must be taken not to further injure the nerve by compressing bone graft material onto the exposed nerve.

Nerve Repositioning

CT imaging and navigation-guided implant placement have provided some protection against IAN injury. However, when preoperative imaging studies indicate that the implants cannot be placed without injury to the nerve, a nerve repositioning procedure may be indicated. In this procedure the lateral cortex of the mandible is removed at the desired location. The MN can be freed from the foramen if the implants are planned in proximity to this area. If necessary, the incisive nerve is transected at its junction with the MN to allow lateralization of the IAN. The nerve is carefully lateralized from the canal to allow placement of the implant(s) medial to the IAC as needed (Fig. 11A–E). An autogenous bone graft, either from the bone removed to unroof the IAC or elsewhere, or bank bone, is always placed between the repositioned nerve and the associated implants to prevent direct contact of the IAN and thermal transmission with the implant(s). Also, artificial

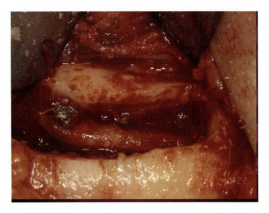

Fig. 9. Exploration of the IAN via a transcutaneous approach and removal of the buccal cortex. A mandibular implant is impinging and deforming the integrity of the nerve.

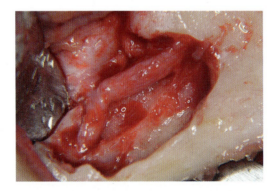

Fig. 10. Exploration of the IAN revealing extensive scar tissue formation compromising the integrity of the nerve secondary to a direct drill injury. The patient presented with pain and anesthesia of the right lower lip and gingiva.

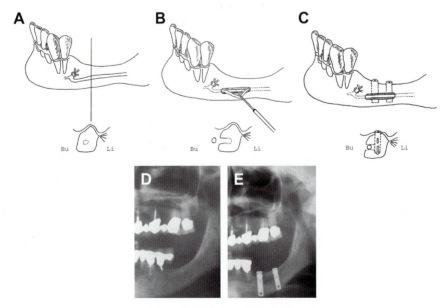

Fig. 11. (*A*) Anticipated implant placement in the posterior right mandible. (*B*) IAN lateralization. (*C*) Placement of 2 dental implants beyond the IAC. (*D*) Preoperative panoramic radiograph of failing dental fixed prosthesis and edentulous posterior mandible. (*E*) Placement of 2 dental implants beyond the IAC after nerve lateralization.

material, such as calcium hydroxyapatite, should never be placed in direct contact with the nerve. A severe inflammatory reaction in the nerve, likened to a chemical burn with dense scarring, accompanied by considerable pain, is often the unfortunate result. Surgical treatment of such injuries is problematic.

Excision of Neuroma

Neuroma formation can be the result of direct drill injury or direct or indirect implant injury to the IAN (Fig. 12A). The neuroma in continuity usually represents a partial transection with subsequent healing predominated by scar and nonconducting nerve tissue. Most of these injuries are repaired using nerve grafts (see below) to restore the continuity of the defect (see Fig. 12B).

External Decompression and Internal Neurolysis

Compression of the IAN can be seen with collapse of the IAC, impingement of the nerve by the implant or other foreign bodies (bone grafting material). External decompression is the removal of surrounding bony, soft tissue structures, and/or foreign material around the nerve (see Fig. 8A). In cases where the implant is found to compress the nerve (see Fig. 9), repositioning of the nerve is considered (see previous section). Internal neurolysis is the opening of the epineurium to inspect the internal nerve structure and decompress the nerve fascicles (see Fig. 8B). If there is a discontinuity defect of 1 or more of the fascicles, then neurorrhaphy or nerve graft reconstruction is indicated. If the nerve is found to be intact, an external decompression and internal neurolysis are sufficient.

Neurorrhaphy

Unlike the LN, injuries to the IAN are difficult to repair by direct neurorrhaphy because of relative inability to advance the IAN to approximation across a nerve gap without tension, unless the incisive nerve (IN) is transected. However, release of the IN leaves the patient with sensory loss in the lower incisor teeth and the mandibular labial gingiva. The stump of the transected IN may develop a stump neuroma, with potential for neuropathic pain. These disadvantages may contraindicate attempts to approximate the IAN without interposition of an autogenous nerve graft.

Nerve Grafts

The sine qua non of a successful neurorrhaphy is to bring the proximal and distal stumps of a transected nerve together and suture them in this position without tension. When the surgeon is unable to accomplish this, reconstruction of the space between the 2 nerve stumps (the nerve gap) can be done with an interpositional nerve graft. Both autologous and allogenic nerve grafts are can be used. The sural (SN) and greater auricular nerve (GAN) are the most commonly used autogenous grafts for maxillofacial nerve repairs (Fig. 13A, B). The SN provides a better size match and longer length. The disadvantages of this graft are the vertical scar just posterior and superior to the lateral malleolus of the ankle, the added operative time to reposition the patient and access a distant surgical

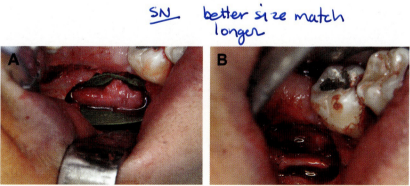

Fig. 12. (*A*) Intraoral exposure of the IAN with a neuroma in continuity secondary to dental implant placement in the area of the second molar. (*B*) Microsurgical repair using an autogenous nerve graft.

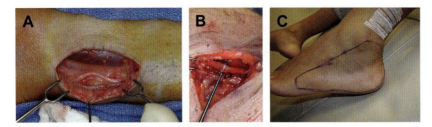

Fig. 13. (*A*) Sural nerve graft harvest. (*B*) GAN harvest. (*C*) Resulting area of anesthesia from a sural nerve harvest.

site, and the associated donor site morbidity (anesthesia of the lateral foot, temporary gait disturbance, pain) (see Fig. 13C). The GAN is easily harvested along its superficial course lateral to the sternocleidomastoid muscle approximately 6 cm inferior to the ear lobe. The main disadvantages of the GAN are the neck scar, ear lobe anesthesia, and its sometimes smaller (than the recipient IAN or LN) diameter. The incision for harvesting the GAN is usually made in a natural skin crease in the lateral neck, and a careful closure usually results in an inconspicuous scar (Fig. 14). Loss of sensation in the lower part of the earlobe is seldom a concern to patients. When the diameter of the GAN is smaller than that of the recipient nerve, a cable graft corrects this discrepancy.

Decellularized human nerve grafts (Axogen, Alachua, FL, USA) are currently readily available for trigeminal nerve reconstruction (see Fig. 8G). Ongoing studies to determine the success of this nerve in the maxillofacial area are pending, although the initial results are promising.

Complications of surgical treatment

The main complications associated with microsurgical repair of nerve injuries from dental implants are related to the type of surgical access to the IAN, sensory outcome, time of surgery, patient age and medical status, and risks of general anesthesia.

Specific Procedure

Surgical access to the IAN is dependent on the location of the nerve injury, the planned procedure, and surgeon's preference. The IAN has a long course, branching from the mandibular nerve in the pterygomandibular space, traveling anteriorly until it enters the mandibular foramen on the medial mandible, continuing within the IAC, and, just before exiting at the mental foramen, dividing into its 2 terminal branches, the IN and the MN. Injuries to the IAN at the mandibular foramen and more proximally in the pterygomandibular space (needle injuries) are difficult to visualize and repair without performing a mandibular ramus osteotomy for additional access. Such operations are seldom done for nerve repair unless as part of tumor resection. However, when the proximal IAN is not accessible or otherwise unrepairable, a nerve-sharing procedure can be done without the requirement of

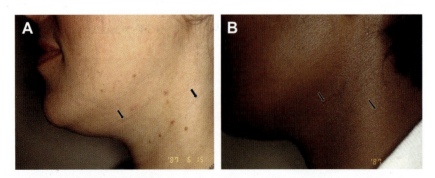

Fig. 14. (*A*) One-year postoperative view of a transcutaneous (Risdon) incision (*left arrow*) and an upper neck incision (*right arrow*) in an 18-year-old white female demonstrating minimal scar visibility. (*B*) Surgical scars (*arrows*) from submandibular incision to expose the IAN and neck incision to harvest a great auricular nerve graft in a 21-year-old African American 1 year after operation.

a mandibular ramus osteotomy. In this operation, an autogenous sural nerve graft is used to connect the proximal GAN to the distal IAN. The authors have used this method to repair the IAN and the LN with success. The IAN at the area of the third molar can be accessed via both intraoral and transcutaneous incisions. The standard Risdon incision allows excellent access to the entire nerve from the area of the mandibular canal to the mental foramen. The main disadvantage of this access is the small possibility of permanent injury to the mandibular branch of the facial nerve (<1% in our experience) and the scar (especially in younger individuals who do not have a naturally visible neck crease). However, placement of the incision along the relaxed skin tension lines, meticulous attention to closure, continued support of the healing incision with adhesive strips, proper skin care, and protection with sunscreens for up to 1 year after operation enhance the likelihood of an inconspicuous scar (see Fig. 14A). In African Americans, the injection of the incision margins with triamcinolone before closure, and on a monthly basis thereafter as indicated, reduces the risk of a hypertrophic scar or keloid (see Fig. 14B).

The IAN can also be exposed transorally by a variety of techniques including a modified sagittal split ramus osteotomy or by decortication (removal of the lateral cortex to create a window of exposure) (Fig. 15). The main disadvantages of the transoral approach are the reduced visibility and access, mainly posterior to the mandibular first molar. Although technically more difficult, successful nerve repairs including interpositional grafting can be done using this approach.

Sensory Outcome

The success of microsurgical repair for restoration of sensory function and elimination of pain is well established. However, as in all operations on sensory nerves, the failure to improve sensation or relieve dysesthesia occurs in some patients. In our study of 186 patients who underwent IAN repair and returned for at least 1 year follow-up, most patients complained preoperatively of numbness (n = 62, 33.3%) or numbness with pain (n = 91, 48.9%). Recovery from neurosensory dysfunction of the IAN (defined by the Medical Research Council Scale [MRSC] as ranging from useful sensory function to complete return of sensation) was achieved in 152 IANs (81.7% with complete recovery or recovery to useful sensory function), whereas 18.3% of nerves showed no or inadequate improvement. For discussion of the MRSC in assessing recovery of sensory nerve injuries, the reader is referred to the paper by Meyer and Rath in further readings.

Time of Surgery, Age of Patient, and Outcome

The results of microsurgical intervention are related statistically to the length of time between nerve injury and microsurgical repair, as shown in our previous studies. In our report of 222 repaired LN injuries, using the logistic regression model, the shorter the duration of time (in months) between nerve injury and repair, the higher the odds of improvement. The likelihood of improvement decreased by 5.8% with each month that passed following injury. The patients who waited more than 9 months for repair were at significantly greater risk for nonimprovement. Likewise, statistical significance was observed between patient age and outcome, representing a 5.5% decrease in chance

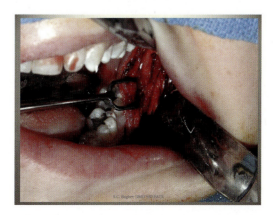

Fig. 15. Exposure of the IAN via an intraoral access.

of recovery for every year of age in patients 45 years and older. Similarly, in our series or 186 IAN repairs (pending publication), the likelihood of functional sensory recovery decreased with increasing duration from nerve injury to its repair, and favorable surgical outcome was decreased with increased age of the patient.

The significance of age and length of time from nerve injury to its repair is especially pertinent to the dental implant patient. In our experience, most of the patients referred to us for evaluation of dental implant-associated nerve injuries were more than 50 years of age and had suffered their nerve injury more than 9 months before our initial consultation.

Patient's Medical Status and Risk of General Anesthesia

Preoperative evaluation of the patient's medical status and risk assessment for general anesthesia for a microneurosurgical operation is performed as needed in consultation with other medical specialties. The risks of general anesthesia for a prolonged procedure include deep vein thrombosis with potential for embolization, pulmonary atelectasis with development of pneumonitis, and urinary tract infection from catheterization. Measures to prevent these risks are part of our routine care of the patient.

Postoperative rehabilitation

Care of the nerve-injured patient does not end with the operation, provision of the usual pain relief, attention to incision care, and recommendations for resumption of normal activities and diet. Measures to enhance sensation and restore related orofacial functions must be included in the rehabilitation of the nerve-injured patient to achieve optimal results.

Younger individuals have better functional recovery after peripheral nerve injury than mature adults. Observations in the human patient are limited, but clinical experience indicates that the efficiency of regeneration is less in later life. Neuropsychological factors also influence the ability of the patient to recovery successfully from a peripheral nerve injury following its surgical repair. There is the need to learn new axonal connections with referral of sensory input to different areas of the central nervous system (CNS). Early in the recovery process, axons exhibit slower conduction time making interpretation more difficult for the CNS until accommodations can be achieved, a situation analogous to a baseball batter having to adjust to a change-up (dramatically slower speed) pitch. Although the older patient is slower to adapt to these changes imposed by recovery from a peripheral nerve injury, neuroplasticity (the ability of the brain to adapt) is still viable even into advanced age.

The concept of sensory reeducation, first developed by Wynn Parry for rehabilitation of hand and upper extremity injuries, has been modified for the maxillofacial regions and shown to be successful in improving sensory function, once responses to pain and static light touch have returned. The goals of sensory reeducation for peripheral trigeminal nerve injuries are to improve or resolve synesthesia (failure to recognize the location of a stimulus), decrease hyperesthesia, improve recognition of the character and amplitude of stimuli (eg, moving or stationary, sharp or dull, light or forceful application, size of area of contact), and decrease subjective differences (eg, numbness) between the affected area and the corresponding normal contralateral area. Following microneurosurgery, we initiate sensory reeducation exercises as soon as the area supplied by the repaired nerve begins to respond to painful stimuli and static light tough (usually within 3–6 months after surgery). The exercises are performed by the patient several times daily for a minimum of 12 months, or longer as needed. During this time the patient is monitored with NST to assess progress. We believe that sensory reeducation contributes to the nerve-injured patient's ability to improve their level of sensory function and associated orofacial activities.

Summary

Treatment of the patient who has sustained a nerve injury from dental implant procedures involves prompt recognition of this complication, evaluation of sensory dysfunction, the position of the nerve vis-à-vis the implant, and timely management of the injured nerve. In some patients, removal or repositioning of the implant and surgical exploration and repair of the injured nerve will maximize the implant patient's potential for a successful recovery from nerve injury.

Further readings

Al-Bishri A, Dahlin L, Sunzel B, et al. Systemic betamethasone accelerates functional recovery after a crush injury to rat sciatic nerve. J Oral Maxillofac Surg 2005;63:973.

Bagheri SC, Meyer RA, Cho S, et al. A retrospective review of microsurgical repair of 186 inferior alveolar nerve injuries. J Oral Maxillofac Surg 2010;68(Suppl 1):27.

Bagheri SC, Meyer RA, Khan HA, et al. Microsurgical repair of peripheral trigeminal nerve injuries from maxillofacial trauma. J Oral Maxillofac Surg 2009;67:1791.

Bagheri SC, Meyer RA, Khan HA, et al. Retrospective review of microsurgical repair of 222 lingual nerve injuries. J Oral Maxillofac Surg 2010;68(4):715–23.

Chaushu G, Taicher S, Haiamish-Shani T, et al. Medicolegal aspects of altered sensation following implant placement in the mandible. Int J Oral Maxillofac Implants 2002;17:413–5.

Gregg JM, Zuniga JR. An outcome analysis of clinical trials of the surgical treatment of traumatic trigeminal sensory neuropathy. Oral Maxillofac Surg Clin North Am 2001;13:377.

LaBanc JP, Van Boven RW. Surgical management of inferior alveolar nerve injuries. Oral Maxillofac Surg Clin North Am 1992;4:425.

Meyer RA. Applications of microneurosurgery to the repair of trigeminal nerve injuries. Oral Maxillofac Surg Clin North Am 1992;4:405.

Meyer RA, Rath EM. Sensory rehabilitation after trigeminal nerve injury or nerve repair. Oral Maxillofac Surg Clin North Am 2001;13:365.

Meyer RA, Ruggiero SL. Guidelines for diagnosis and treatment of peripheral trigeminal nerve injuries. Oral Maxillofac Surg Clin North Am 2001;13:383.

Meyer RA. Nerve harvesting procedures. Atlas Oral Maxillofac Surg Clin North Am 2001;9:77.

Pogrel MA, Bryan J, Regezi J. Nerve damage associated with inferior alveolar nerve blocks. J Am Dent Assoc 1995;126(8):1150–5.

Pogrel MA, Thamby S. Permanent nerve involvement resulting from inferior alveolar nerve blocks. J Am Dent Assoc 2000;131(7):901–7.

Pogrel MA. The results of microneurosurgery of the inferior alveolar and lingual nerve. J Oral Maxillofac Surg 2002;60:485.

Pola R, Aprahamian TR, Bosch-Marce M, et al. Age-dependent VEGF expression and intraneural neovascularization during regeneration of peripheral nerves. Neurobiol Aging 2004;25:1361.

Seddon HJ. Nerve lesions complicating certain closed bone injuries. J Am Med Assoc 1947;135:691.

Seo K, Tanaka Y, Terumitsu M, et al. Efficacy of steroid treatment for sensory impairment after orthognathic surgery. J Oral Maxillofac Surg 2004;62:1193.

Susarla S, Kaban L, Donoff RB, et al. Does early repair of lingual nerve injuries improve functional sensory recovery? J Oral Maxillofac Surg 2007;65:1070–6.

Verdu E, Ceballos D, Vilches JJ, et al. Influence of aging on peripheral nerve function and regeneration. J Peripher Nerv Syst 2000;5:191.

Wynn Parry CB. Brachial plexus injuries. Br J Hosp Med 1984;32(3):130–2, 134–9.

Ziccardi V, Steinberg M. Timing of trigeminal nerve microsurgery: a review of the literature. J Oral Maxillofac Surg 2007;65:1341–5.

Nerve Injuries from Mandibular Third Molar Removal

Roger A. Meyer, DDS, MS, MD[a,*], Shahrokh C. Bagheri, DMD, MD[b,c,d,e]

[a]Maxillofacial Consultants Ltd, 1021 Holt's Ferry, Greensboro, GA 30642, USA
[b]Private Practice, Georgia Oral & Facial Surgery, 1880 West Oak Parkway, Suite 215, Marietta, GA 30062, USA
[c]Division of Oral and Maxillofacial Surgery, Department of Surgery, Northside Hospital, 1000 Johnson Ferry Road, Atlanta, GA 30342, USA
[d]Department of Surgery, School of Medicine, Emory University, 1365 Clifton Road NE, Atlanta, GA 30322, USA
[e]Department of Oral & Maxillofacial Surgery, School of Dentistry, Medical College of Georgia, 1120 15th Street, Augusta, GA 30912, USA

In surveys of oral and maxillofacial surgery practice, removal of teeth is the most frequently performed operation. Removal of an impacted mandibular third molar tooth (M3) presents unique surgical challenges. One such challenge is the risk of injury to the peripheral branches of the trigeminal nerve, which provide sensation to the oral and facial regions. Indeed, in the practice of oral and maxillofacial surgery, because of their unfavorable effects on orofacial sensation and related functions (such as eating, drinking, washing, speaking, shaving, kissing), nerve injuries are currently the most frequent cause of litigation against oral and maxillofacial surgeons (OMFSs) in the United States. Since the seminal work of Merrill in the 1960s to 1970s on the injury, pathophysiology, and repair of inferior alveolar and lingual nerve (LN) injuries, much research and clinical work has been directed toward the prevention and treatment of peripheral trigeminal nerve injuries.

During the removal of an M3, the inferior alveolar nerve (IAN), lying adjacent to M3's roots, and the LN, often located just medial to M3's crown at or near the mandibular lingual alveolar crestal bone, are at risk of injury from the various surgical maneuvers composing the operation. Such injuries may not resolve in a reasonable period but instead persist and result in significant permanent sensory dysfunction in the distribution of the involved nerve. On the other hand, the long buccal nerve (LBN) is frequently knowingly transected during the standard incision for exposure of the M3, but only rarely does this maneuver cause bothersome sensory aberration (Fig. 1).

Nerve injury is a known and accepted risk of the removal of M3s and it may occur despite the best of care. Proactive measures during evaluation and removal of M3s may reduce the incidence of nerve injury and the disturbance of sensory alteration. When nerve injury caused by the removal of an M3 fails to resolve promptly and the resulting paresthesias and/or dysesthesias are unacceptable to the patient, timely treatment gives the patient the best chance of a favorable outcome.

Incidence

Various retrospective reports from individual surgical practices in the literature have given only a limited sample of the incidence or frequency of nerve injuries related to removal of M3s. From this information it had been estimated that a temporary injury to the IAN or LN occurred in 1.0% to 4.4% of patients, with 0.1% to 1.0% of the injuries failing to resolve and becoming permanent in the absence of treatment. New data in 2005 obtained from 535 responses (95% of membership) in

---

The authors dedicate this article to Ralph George Merrill, DDS, MScD, former Chairman (1969–1997), Department of Oral and Maxillofacial Surgery, Oregon Health and Sciences University, Portland, whose research, writing, teaching, mentoring, and surgical skills in the field of peripheral nerve injuries have been a constant inspiration.

* Corresponding author. 1021 Holt's Ferry, Greensboro, GA 30642.
E-mail address: rameyer@aol.com

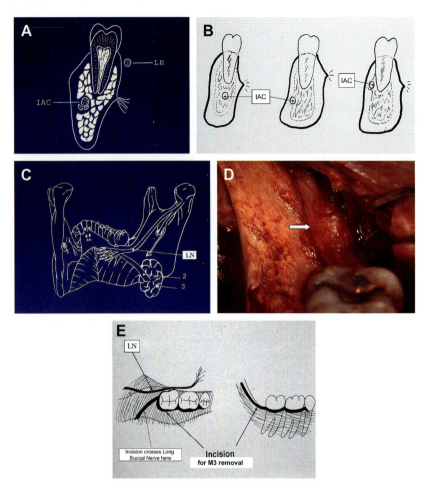

Fig. 1. Anatomic relationships of LN, IAN, and LBN. (*A*) The usual or classic positions of LN and IAN. (*B*) Variations in the location of IAC, based on the authors' experience in exposing the IAN for microsurgical repair. (*C*) One of the 3 described locations of the LN at or near the alveolar crest on the medial surface of the posterior mandible area places it at risk during M3 removal. 2, submandibular salivary duct; 3, submandibular salivary gland. (*D*) The LN (*arrow*), exposed during dissection in preparation for a sagittal split osteotomy of the right mandibular ramus, is seen located superior to the alveolar crest. (*E*) The incision for raising a mucoperiosteal flap to gain access to an impacted M3 usually crosses the path of the LBN. Significant sensory dysfunction of the LBN is extremely rare following M3 removal. IAC, inferior alveolar canal.

a survey of the California Association of Oral and Maxillofacial Surgeons have provided a more comprehensive view of this problem. In 95% of surgeons' practices, 1 or more patients per year sustained an IAN injury (78% of the injuries were classified as permanent), whereas 1 or more LN injuries were reported in 53% of practices (46% of the injuries deemed permanent). Mean rates for all injuries per thousand M3s removed were 0.4% for IAN injuries (4/1000) and 0.01% for LN injury (1/1000), whereas the permanent injury rates were 0.04% (1/2500) for the IAN and 0.010% (1/10,000) for the LN. The cause of IAN injury was known (although not specified) in 261 respondents; on the other hand, only 31 surgeons knew the cause of LN injury. This may be because of the visualization of the IAN in the depths of an M3 socket after tooth removal, whereas the LN is often contained within the lingual soft tissue flap and could not be directly observed by the surgeon. Unsurprisingly, injury rates by surgeons were lower among those surgeons performing greater numbers of extractions per year (range, 100–2000) and having more years of experience.

Not all M3s are removed by specialists. No recent hard data are available for nerve injury complication rates among general dental practitioners (GDPs) who remove M3s. At present, it is estimated that approximately 50% of M3s are extracted by GDPs in the United States. In the authors' combined clinical experience of more than 40 years of caring for nerve injuries, the number of nerve injury referrals from OMFSs and GDPs are approximately equal. However, there may be a bias in that GDPs tend to do the easier cases and refer all others to OMFSs, including those with higher known risk of nerve injury (ie, proximity of M3 roots to inferior alveolar canal [IAC] as seen on a radiograph).

Cause

Removal of M3s is the procedure most frequently associated with nerve injuries in oral and maxillofacial surgery practice (Box 1). However, the exact cause of nerve injury is frequently not known, especially if the involved nerve is not directly visualized during removal of M3s. Indirect deduction from imaging studies on the relationship of the tooth roots to the IAC provides indicators of likelihood of injury to IAN. Because the LN resides in soft tissue and most preoperative evaluations for M3 removal do not include imaging with MRI, no data exist to guide the clinician on estimating the LN position or risk of injury. (See the article by Miloro in this issue for further exploration of this topic.)

Speculation on the cause of nerve injury in a given patient is often a reflection of whether the discussant is the surgeon (unexpected or rare anatomic variation, unavoidable mishap despite the best of care) or a disgruntled patient (error in surgeon's technique, not adhering to a standard procedure). From the authors' personal experience in the removal of M3s and in caring for patients referred for nerve injury treatment, several aspects of the operation for M3 removal seem, either by inference or direct observation, to pose a risk for injury to the IAN, LN, or LBN. These maneuvers include injection of a local anesthetic, location of the incision, retraction of a soft tissue flap for access to the tooth, removal of associated soft tissue pathology (eg, enlarged follicular sac or cyst, periapical inflammatory/granulation tissue), removal of bone, tooth sectioning, suturing, and administration of medications (either after removal of the tooth [ie, antibiotic] or in the postoperative period for treatment of alveolar osteitis [dry socket]). Whether these risk factors can be overcome by proactive modification of techniques or procedures is a matter of conjecture in any given patient. However, each of these risk factors is discussed in the following section, along with suggestions for the reduction of the risk of nerve injury.

Prevention

It may or may not be possible to reduce the number of risk factors for nerve injury during the removal of M3. However, even in an operation that meets all standards of care and is performed by a well-trained and experienced OMFS, it is known and accepted that risks and complications can still and do occur. The following suggestions are presented without certainty as to their success in minimizing the risk of nerve injury.

Imaging Studies

Imaging studies are the basis for evaluation of contemplated M3 removal. An adequate radiograph should display the entire tooth, surrounding bone, periapical region, and IAC. This visualization may be possible with a periapical film, but a panoramic view is most commonly used as a basic imaging study (Fig. 2). In addition to the depth of M3 within the mandible (soft tissue, partial bone, and complete bone impaction), and the angulation of the tooth within the alveolar bone (vertical,

---

Box 1. Procedures associated with peripheral trigeminal nerve injuries are listed in descending order of frequency, based on the authors' combined experience (1981 to 2010)

- Removal of lower third molar teeth
- Orthognathic surgery
- Maxillofacial trauma (fractures, soft tissue injury, gunshot wound)
- Dental implants
- Cyst or tumor excision
- Preprosthetic surgery (vestibuloplasty, ridge augmentation)
- Root canal treatment (canal filling, apical surgery)
- Local anesthetic injection
- Salivary gland excision
- Biopsy

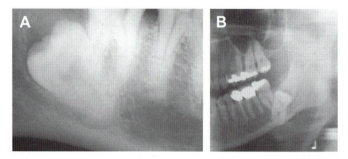

Fig. 2. Plain radiographic views of M3s. (*A*) An adequate periapical plain film shows the entire tooth and its relationship with the IAC. (*B*) Panoramic plain film showing unusual position of M3 at the inferior border of mandible. (*B, From* Freedman GL. Intentional partial odontectomy: report of case. J Oral Maxillofac Surg 1992;50:419; with permission.)

horizontal, mesioangular, distoangular), perhaps, the most important information is the position of the tooth roots in relation to the IAC. In determining this relationship from a plain radiograph, which shows overlap of the IAC and the tooth roots, 2 factors are assessed: (1) the *radiodensity of the root* where it is overlaid by the IAC and (2) the *width (diameter) of the IAC* as it crosses over the roots. Four conditions can be identified: (1) *superimposition*, in which the roots and IAC are overlaid in the 2-dimensional radiograph but are actually not in physical contact or proximity; (2) *notching* of the root, in which the IAC is in intimate physical contact within an indentation in the side of the root; (3) *grooving*, in which the IAC is in intimate contact within a concave defect in the apex of the root; and (4) *perforation*, in which the IAC actually penetrates through the root (Fig. 3). There will be little or no loss of radiodensity of the root, which is superimposed on the IAC as seen in a plain radiograph, but is not in actual contact. When the root has been notched, grooved, or penetrated by the IAC, however, there will be a definite line of demarcation indicating a change in root radiodensity. Additionally, when the IAC penetrates the M3 root, the IAC width (diameter) generally narrows noticeably. Conditions other than superimposition might require further evaluation with a computed tomographic scan (Fig. 4). Documentation of notching, grooving, or penetration of the root may

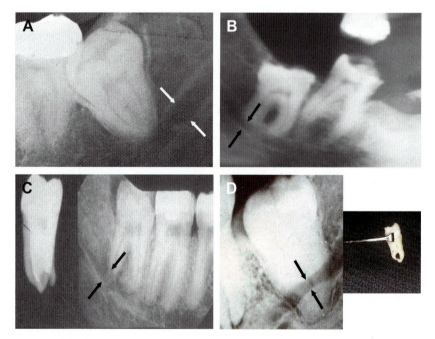

Fig. 3. Determining the relationship of M3 and IAC from plain radiographs. (*A*) Superimposition of M3 and IAC. There is neither a line of demarcation nor a change of radiodensity of M3 roots where they are crossed by IAC, and the diameter of IAC (*arrows*) does not narrow in that area. (*B*) Notching of M3 by IAC. There is a definite line of demarcation and loss of radiodensity of the M3 roots where crossed by IAC (*arrows*). (*C*) Grooving of the apex of M3 by IAC. There is a definite line of demarcation and loss of radiodensity of the distal root of M3 where crossed by IAC (*arrows*). (*D*) Penetration of M3 root. There is a definite line of demarcation and loss of radiodensity of M3 where crossed by IAC, and the diameter of IAC (*arrows*) narrows.

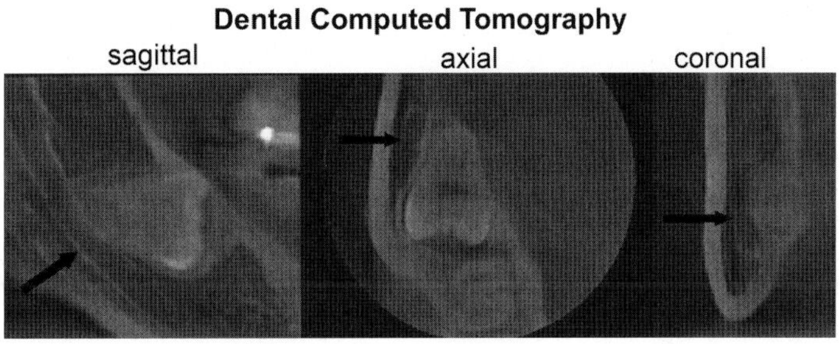

Dental Computed Tomography

sagittal   axial   coronal

Fig. 4. Use of computed tomography to determine the exact location of M3 and IAC (*arrows*). Multiple orientations (sagittal, axial, coronal) give exact information to assist the clinician in decisions regarding planning for partial or complete M3 removal. (*From* Hatano Y, Kurita K, Kuroiwa Y, et al. Clinical evaluations of coronectomy (intentional partial odontectomy) for mandibular third molars using dental computed tomography: a case-control study. J Oral Maxillofac Surg 2009;67:1810; with permission.)

be an indication to perform subtotal removal of the tooth, avoiding the portion of the root that is in intimate contact with the IAC (see Coronectomy under Treatment).

Injection of a Local Anesthetic

Injection of a local anesthetic into the pterygomandibular space for operative anesthesia of the IAN, LBN, and LN and early postoperative pain control is most often done after the patient is under intravenous sedation or general anesthesia. Therefore, the paresthesia (sudden shocking sensation, often with radiation of pain to the teeth, jaw, lower lip, or tongue) that might occur if the injection needle contacts the nerve is not observed. However, if the usual preinjection aspiration returns blood into the anesthetic carpule, it can be assumed that the needle has contacted the IAN and/or LN. Before proceeding with the injection, the needle should be withdrawn 2 to 3 mm, and then the aspiration is repeated. If no blood returns into the carpule, the injection can proceed. When a conscious patient notes a paresthesia, the same routine of slight withdrawal of the needle and aspiration before proceeding is done. The incident is noted in the patient's record, and a follow-up evaluation of sensory function is done at the first postoperative visit (see the article by Meyer and Bagheri elsewhere in this issue for further exploration of this topic).

Soft Tissue Incision

A correctly placed soft tissue incision avoids trauma to the LN (Fig. 5). The posterolateral extension of the incision routinely crosses the path of the LBN (see Fig. 1E) making trauma to this nerve virtually inevitable. However, significant sensory dysfunction of the LBN is extremely rare (see Treatment).

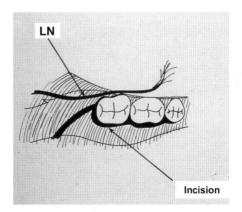

Fig. 5. Incision for exposure of M3 is placed in buccal gingival sulcus of erupted molars, then extended from the distobuccal corner of the last erupted molar lateroposteriorly to avoid intersection with the LN.

Soft Tissue Flap Retraction

Soft tissue flap retraction affords not only access to and visualization of the surgical field but also protection to important adjacent soft tissue structures, including the LN (Fig. 6). Although retraction of the lingual flap might result in an increased incidence of temporary paresthesia of the LN, the retracting instrument serves as a protective shield should an osteotome, an elevator, or a high-speed rotating burr penetrate the lingual bone and otherwise possibly produce a serious injury of the LN.

Removing Soft Tissue Pathology

Care is taken in removing soft tissue pathology (eg, enlarged follicular sac or dentigerous cyst) from around the crown of the tooth, especially if the lingual bone has been perforated by erosive force of the cyst lest the LN be in jeopardy (Fig. 7). Likewise, curettage of apical inflammatory/granulation tissue should be done with care when the IAN is known to be adjacent.

Bone Removal

Whether bone removal is done with osteotomes or high-speed rotating burs, care must be taken to avoid, if possible, perforation of the lingual alveolar bone (Fig. 8). If perforation does occur, a properly placed retractor serves as a protective shield for the LN.

Sectioning Teeth

When sectioning teeth, the burr should be brought three-fourths of the way through; then, an elevator should be used to complete separation of the tooth segment, thus avoiding direct trauma to the LN or IAN (Fig. 9).

Partial Odontectomy

If the roots lie in intimate contact with the IAC, a partial odontectomy (coronectomy) should be considered. The roots left in situ may remain in place and rarely, if ever, cause infection or other untoward incident (Fig. 10). In some cases, the roots migrate in a superior direction away from the IAC, allowing their subsequent removal to be nonproblematic (Fig. 11).

Medicating the Socket

Medicating the socket with antibiotic cones or powder at the conclusion of tooth removal or postoperation with analgesic liquids or pastes to relieve alveolar osteitis is inadvisable if either the LN or IAC contents were directly exposed/visualized during the operation. Such medications might cause a chemical burn when they are in direct contact with or able to percolate toward the nerve.

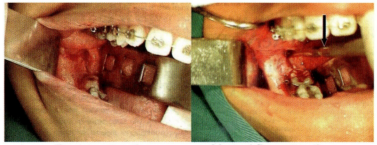

Fig. 6. Tongue retractor in place at the beginning of operation for removal of M3 (*left*). Lingual mucoperiosteal flap has been raised and is held by an additional instrument (eg, Henahan, Freer, or Seldin retractor *arrow*) to afford protection to the underlying LN (*right*). (*From* Gomes AC, Vasconcelos BC, Silva ED, et al. Lingual nerve damage after mandibular third molar surgery: a randomized clinical trial. J Oral Maxillofac Surg 2005;63:1444; with permission.)

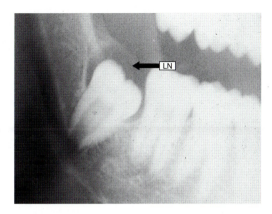

Fig. 7. M3 with enlarged follicular sac or early dentigerous cyst, which has eroded lingual alveolar bone. During removal of soft tissue surrounding M3 crown, surgeon inadvertently removed a portion of the adjacent LN (contained in tissue specimen sent to pathologist, interpreted as "follicular sac and associated granulation tissue, also containing nerve"). The patient had sustained a discontinuity defect of the right LN and required a microsurgical repair (neurorrhaphy), which resulted in nearly total return of sensation to the right tongue and lingual gingival (S3+) after 1 year.

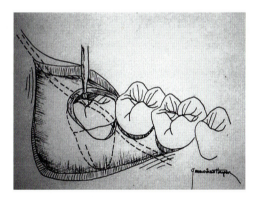

Fig. 8. When removing bone to provide access to and exposure of M3, care is taken to avoid penetrating the lingual alveolar bone. If lingual bone must be removed to deliver the tooth, the lingual soft tissues (including LN) are protected with a suitable retractor (see Fig. 6). (*From* Merrill RG. Prevention, treatment and prognosis for nerve injury related to the difficult impaction. Dent Clin North Am 1979;23:471; with permission.)

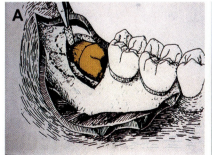 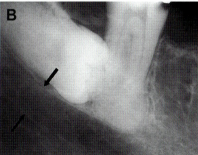

Fig. 9. Tooth sectioning. (*A*) When the M3 must be sectioned using a high-speed drill, carry the bur only three-fourth of the way through the tooth structure before separating the crown or the roots with an elevator. (*B*) The IAC (*arrows*) often lurks just beneath a deeply imbedded horizontally affected M3.

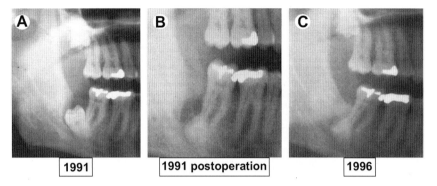

Fig. 10. Planned partial odontectomy (coronectomy). (*A*) Preoperative view of distoangular M3 lying adjacent to IAC. (*B*) Immediate postoperative film showing removal of M3 crown; roots left in situ to avoid injury to IAN. (*C*) After 5 years, regeneration of bone and no reaction around retained M3 roots are noticed. (*From* Freedman GL. Intentional partial odontectomy: review of cases. J Oral Maxillofac Surg 1997;55:524; with permission.)

Placing Sutures

When placing sutures, especially when lingual bone has been eroded by pathology, fractured off with an ankylosed tooth segment, or removed by instrumentation, avoid too large a bite of the lingual soft tissue flap with the suture needle lest the LN be impaled (Fig. 12).

Evaluation

Management of a nerve injury when it does occur during removal of M3s requires prompt recognition of the problem (either by direct visualization during the operation or at the first postoperative visit when the patient presents the complaint), a standardized examination including neurosensory testing (NST) and an appropriate and timely plan of treatment. For a comprehensive discussion of this subject, please see the article by Meyer and Bagheri elsewhere in this issue.

Treatment

Timing is critical in the treatment of nerve injuries. Following nerve damage or severance there is a progression of events, collectively termed Wallerian degeneration, in which the axons distal to the

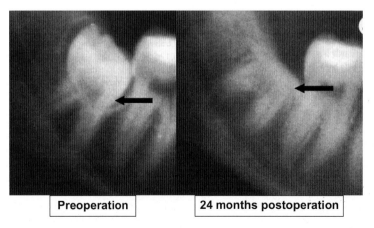

Fig. 11. Root migration after intention coronectomy. Roots of M3 rest on IAC. Arrow indicates cemento-enamel junction (CEJ) of M3 (*left*). Two years following M3 coronectomy, the remaining tooth fragment has migrated occlusally (*arrow* indicates CEJ). (*From* Dolanmaz D, Yildrim G, Isik K, et al. A preferable technique for protecting the inferior alveolar nerve: coronectomy. J Oral Maxillofac Surg 2009;67:1236; with permission.)

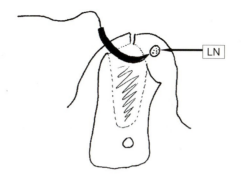

Fig. 12. When closing the incision after M3 removal, look for LN before placing needle through lingual soft tissue flap. (*Data from* Goldberg MH. Frequency of trigeminal nerve injury following third molar removal [letter]. J Oral Maxillofac Surg 2005;63:1783.)

injury site undergo necrosis and phagocytosis. The nerve cell body enlarges and increases metabolic activity as it attempts to produce new axonal growth. After phagocytosis of distal axons is complete, new proximal axonal sprouts begin to attempt to grow across the injury gap, recannulate the distal nerve endoneurial tubules, and extend to neural end plates in the mucosal or skin surface. At the same time, those endoneurial tubules that lack axonal recannulation begin to collapse, one by one, and become replaced with scar tissue. When a critical mass of endoneurial tubules becomes irretrievably lost to recannulation, the nerve can no longer be expected to recover (Fig. 13). In humans, this process has been estimated to begin at 1 to 2 months after injury and passes a point of no return after 9 to 15 months. Indeed, in the authors' research on the outcomes of nerve injuries, successful repair is most likely if nerves are surgically repaired within 9 months of injury, with progressively decreasing success rates thereafter (Fig. 14). Age of the patient is also important because success rates decline progressively after 45 years of age (Fig. 15).

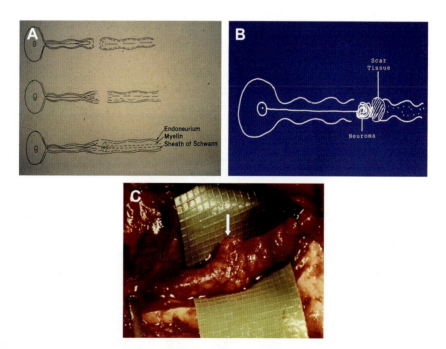

Fig. 13. Wallerian degeneration after sensory nerve injury. (*A*) Nerve has been severed, and necrosis and phagocytosis of distal axons is in progress (to the right of nerve gap) (*top*). Phagocytosis of distal axons completed. New axonal sprouts appear in proximal nerve stump (to the left of nerve gap) (*middle*). Proximal axonal sprouts cross the nerve gap and cannulate distal endoneurial tubules. Axons continue to grow distally toward neural endplates in skin or mucosa (*bottom*). (*B*) Axonal sprouts from proximal nerve stump may encounter an obstacle (ie, scar tissue or foreign body) preventing them from traversing nerve gap and recannulating distal endoneurial tubules. In such instances, the axonal sprouts form a proximal stump neuroma, and the ability of the nerve to conduct impulses (physiologic continuity) is blocked. (*C*) Clinical appearance of a neuroma in continuity (*arrow*) of the IAN. Although the nerve seems to be in anatomic continuity, intervening scar tissue blocks transmission of impulses across the injured area of the IAN.

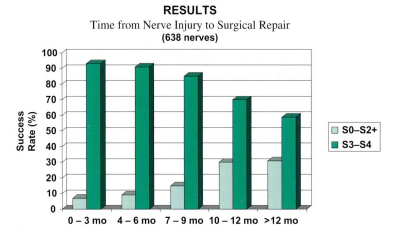

Fig. 14. Effect of time from injury to surgical repair of sensory nerves on outcome. Successful recovery of sensory function (S3–S4) is inversely related to length of time from injury to operation and it becomes significant when the repair is done more than 9 months after nerve injury.

Open Nerve Injuries

Open nerve injuries (directly observed during the operation) can be repaired immediately if the surgeon has microsurgical skills and if general endotracheal anesthesia, capable assistance, and proper instruments are available. Otherwise, the nerve ends are gently placed into appropriate position and tagged with fine nonreactive sutures, if possible. A description of the location and nature of the injury is given in the operative report. Prompt referral is made to a microsurgeon for definitive treatment. During some M3 removals, a root fragment is displaced into the IAC. In general, a surgeon lacking microsurgical skills should not attempt retrieval of the fragment through an extraction socket. It is recommended that the fragment be left in situ, the incident is mentioned in the operative report, and the patient followed up to see if sensory dysfunction develops. In many cases, there is no permanent sensory deficit and no reaction develops around the retained root, making its removal unnecessary (Fig. 16). If a sensory deficit is present at the first postoperative visit, a referral to a microsurgeon could be made.

Occasionally, a surgeon is presented with an emergency referral from a GDP who attempted and failed to complete the removal of an M3 under local anesthesia and asks the surgeon to attend the patient immediately. Of course, the implication is that because the extraction area is still under local

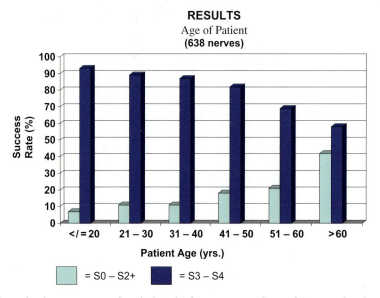

Fig. 15. Effect of age of patient on outcome of surgical repair of sensory nerves. Successful sensory function recovery (S3–S4) is inversely related to patient age and it becomes significant in patients older than 45 years.

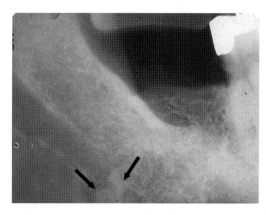

Fig. 16. Radiograph shows M3 root fragments (*arrows*) displaced into IAC several years ago. The patient had a brief period of paresthesia following removal of the tooth, which recovered completely within a few weeks. Note lack of inflammatory reaction in surrounding bone.

anesthesia, the GDP expects the surgeon to remove the remains of the tooth forthwith. There is nothing really emergent (or life threatening) about this situation, but considerable stress may have been generated in both the GDP and the patient. Before proceeding, however, the surgeon is well advised, after explaining the necessity to the patient, to obtain a suitable radiograph of the operative site to identify the location of tooth remnants and to rule out a mandibular fracture (Fig. 17). Furthermore, the surgeon should wait until the local anesthetic has worn off and perform a screening NST to document whether or not the patient has a nerve injury because of the GDP's attempt to remove the tooth. Then, the surgeon can complete the tooth removal with the anesthetic of his/her choice. The only immediate treatment that need be rendered while awaiting the end of local anesthesia is to achieve hemostasis, if bleeding from the operative site is a problem. Because this situation often occurs late in the day, the decision might be made to defer the completion of the extraction to a subsequent day, and in the meantime, the surgeon provides appropriate medications (antibiotics, analgesics) as indicated.

Closed Nerve Injury

The authors have developed an algorithm to provide suggestions for management of the patient who sustains a closed nerve injury (not observed by the surgeon during the operation) during removal of an M3 (day 0) (Fig. 18). When the patient returns for the first postoperative visit, he/she is questioned about any lingering sensory deficit in the areas of distribution of the LN (tongue, lingual gingival, taste sensation), IAN (lower lip, chin, labial gingival), or LBN (posterior buccal gingival, cheek). If the patient presents a sensory complaint, this is evaluated by an examination that includes

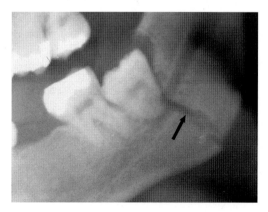

Fig. 17. Patient had a prolonged unsuccessful attempt to remove the left M3 under LA by a GDP, who then referred the patient (while still under LA) to an OMFS for emergency removal. Panoramic film taken by the OMFS before proceeding with M3 removal shows a fracture of the left mandibular angle involving the M3 (*arrow*). After waiting for LA to wear off, the OMFS performed NST, which revealed anesthesia of distribution of left IAN. Patient required open reduction/internal fixation of the fracture and removal of M3. Normal sensory function returned to left IAN within 3 months of injury. No repair of IAN was done. LA, local anesthesia.

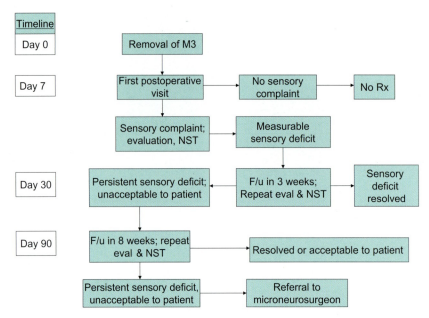

Fig. 18. Algorithm with suggestions for evaluation and management of closed sensory nerve injuries associated with removal of M3s. eval, evaluation; F/u, follow-up; Rx, treatment. (See text for explanation and discussion.)

NST (see the article by Meyer and Bagheri elsewhere in this issue.) If no measurable sensory deficit is found, no further treatment is necessary. If, however, there is a measurable hypoesthesia, anesthesia, or pain response, it is documented in the patient's record, and the patient is scheduled for a subsequent visit at 4 weeks following the date of tooth removal (day 30). At that time, if the sensory complaint has resolved and there are normal responses to NST, no further treatment is indicated. The patient who continues to have sensory complaints and gives abnormal responses to NST is reappointed to be seen in 8 more weeks (day 90). Again, NST is repeated, and if the patient gives normal responses and has no sensory complaint or if the patient considers the sensory deficit acceptable and refuses treatment, the problem is considered to have resolved and no further treatment is scheduled. On the other hand, if the patient's sensory complaints and abnormal responses to NST persist and are unacceptable to the patient, it is considered that the patient has a nerve injury that may require surgical intervention or other specialized treatment. Referral is arranged without further delay for the patient to be seen and evaluated by a microsurgeon capable of performing surgical repair of the injured nerve, if indicated. The importance of decision making regarding treatment at 90 days after the nerve injury deserves attention. In the authors' experience and that of others who care for nerve injuries, patients who remain anesthetic (no responses to NST) in this situation have little or no chance of undergoing spontaneous recovery in the future, so further expectant observation in the vain hope of a late sensory recovery only deprives them of the earliest opportunity for surgical intervention when the chance of a successful outcome is maximized. In addition, patients who may have some responses to NST but whose primary complaint is pain need to be attended early on in their postinjury course by a microsurgeon lest their symptoms progress to a chronic intractable pain syndrome for which any treatment, medical or surgical, becomes problematic.

Peripheral Trigeminal Nerve Injuries

These injuries are repaired (microneurosurgery) under general endotracheal anesthesia in the operating room. The patient must remain totally motionless to facilitate accomplishing delicate procedures on small structures (the LN, IAN, and LBN are generally 1–2 mm in diameter) under magnification with surgical loupes (2.5×–5.0× power) or the operating microscope. The depth of anesthesia is used to control bleeding from the operative site, which facilitates visualization. Strict sterile conditions are necessary when operating outside the oral cavity for submandibular exposure of the IAN or approaching the neck or lower extremity for harvesting a nerve graft. It is not always known in advance of surgical exposure of the injured nerve whether or not an autogenous nerve graft will be required for reconstruction of a nerve gap. The LBN and LN are always approached

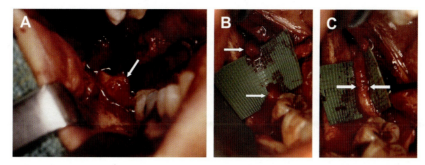

Fig. 19. Transoral exposure of the LN. (*A*) Exploration of an injured right LN with a neuroma in continuity (*arrow*). (*B*) Excision of neuroma creates a nerve gap between the proximal and distal LN stumps (*arrows*). (*C*) After dissection and mobilization of the proximal and distal LN stumps, they are able to be brought together, and a neurorrhaphy is performed without tension (*arrows* indicate suture line).

transorally (see Figs. 1E and 5; Fig. 19). Depending on the location of injury and the access needed for good visualization and performance of the surgical maneuvers, the IAN may be exposed either transorally or transcutaneously (via a submandibular incision) (Fig. 20). Once the nerve is exposed, step-by-step procedures are performed, usually one after the other until the nerve is repaired (Box 2). In the case of a discontinuity defect of the nerve (partial or complete severance), suturing without tension is the sine qua non of a successful nerve repair, whether done by neurorrhaphy or by a nerve grafting procedure. In the authors' experience, most LN discontinuity defects are able to be repaired by neurorrhaphy because the proximal and distal nerve limbs, which often have a curvaceous course within soft tissue, can be mobilized by proximal and distal dissection and when straightened can be brought together easily without tension. On the other hand, IAN injuries that present a discontinuity defect are often difficult to mobilize and advance within the IAC and more likely to require a nerve graft to reconstruct the nerve gap. All the LBN injuries in the authors' small series were discontinuity defects and were treated by excision of a proximal stump neuroma and neurorrhaphy.

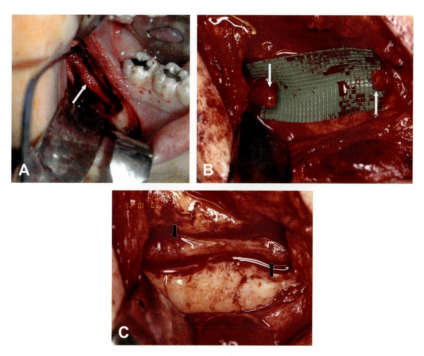

Fig. 20. Surgical approaches to the IAN. (*A*) The IAN (*arrow*) is exposed transorally by unroofing the IAC in the mandibular molar region. It is not always possible to obtain adequate visualization and access for instrumentation required for nerve repair in this area. (*B*) The right IAN has been approached through a submandibular transcutaneous incision, a neuroma has been removed from the proximal nerve stump (*left arrow*), and the proximal and distal nerve stumps (*arrows*) have been debrided in preparation for reconstruction of the nerve gap with an autogenous nerve graft. (*C*) The right IAN has been reconstructed with an autogenous right great auricular nerve graft (suture lines marked by *arrows*). The sural nerve is also a frequent choice as donor nerve.

Box 2. Surgical maneuvers performed sequentially during nerve repair. Surgeon may conclude operation at any step when repair has been successfully completed

- External decompression, removal of bone, scar, foreign body
- Internal neurolysis
- Excision of neuroma, scar tissue
- Mobilization and advancement of nerve stumps
- Approximation of nerve stumps, neurorrhapy without tension
- Reconstruction of nerve gap with nerve graft or alloplastic tube
- Nerve-sharing procedure
- Nerve capping or redirection procedure

Table 1
The MRCS for grading recovery of sensory nerve injuries

Score	Assessment
S0	No recovery
S1	Recovery of deep cutaneous sensation
S2	Return of some superficial pain/tactile sensation
S2+	Same as S2 with hyperesthesia
S3	Same as S2 without hyperesthesia; static 2pd > 15 mm
S3+	Same as S3 with good stimulus localization; 2pd = 7–15 mm
S4	Same as S3+, except 2pd = 2–6 mm

S3 and S3+ denote useful sensory function.
S4 is complete recovery.
Abbreviation: 2pd, 2-point discrimination.
Data from Birch R, Bonney G, Wynn Parry CB. Surgical disorders of the peripheral nerves. Philadelphia: WB Saunders, 1999. p. 235–43.

Table 2
Results of repair of IAN, LN, and LBN that were injured during removal of M3 (based on authors' experience)

Nerve	Number (n)	Success rate (%)[a]
IAN	70	81.7
LN	191	90.5
LBN	4	100.0

[a] Successful recovery following nerve repair: MRCS rating of S3 or S3+ (useful sensory function) or S4 (complete recovery of sensory function).

> **Box 3. Postoperative rehabilitation for the patient with nerve injury may include any or all of the modalities listed**
>
> - Physical therapy
> - Management of pain syndromes
> - Counseling, pyschiatric therapy, support group
> - Restoration of activities of daily living (work, spouse, recreation)
> - Sensory reeducation
> - Maintenance of supportive doctor-patient relationship

The results to be expected from the microsurgical repair of nerve injuries are highly dependent on the surgeon's training and experience. In a review of the authors' nerve injury repairs, results improved with increasing numbers of cases operated. There is estimated to be a threshold number of 50 operations, more than which the surgeon has reached a steady state of predictable results. This number can be accumulated during training, by assisting other surgeons, in the laboratory on animals, and finally in the surgeon's own practice. The authors have completed more than 800 microneurosurgical operations during a combined total of nearly 40 years of experience, with an overall success rate of more than 80% (useful sensory function or better) as determined by the Medical Research Council Scale (MRCS). This scale is a method of assessment for sensory nerve injuries, was originally devised in the United Kingdom for injuries of the hand, and has been successfully adapted to the maxillofacial region (Table 1). A review of results of the authors' microsurgical repair of 265 injuries of the IAN, LN, and LBN sustained during removal of M3s (based on the criteria of the MRCS) is presented in Table 2.

The treatment of the nerve-injured patient is not finished with completion of the microneurosurgery and healing of the incisions. Additional therapy in the postoperative period may include any or all of the following: physical therapy to restore mandibular range of motion or to assist with ambulation when a sural nerve graft is harvested from the lower extremity; management of postnerve injury pain syndromes; counseling, participation in a support group, psychiatric support, and/or restoration of activities of daily living; and sensory reeducation to assist the patient in relearning new nerve connections, localization and characterization of stimuli, maximizing reduction of pain or hypersensitivity, and improving or restoring orofacial functions (Box 3). Some of this care may be provided in multispecialty clinics, especially if the patient's predominant postnerve injury complaint continues to be pain. Postoperative treatment may continue for 1 or more years after nerve repair and is based on the establishment and continuance of a close and supportive relationship of the surgeon with the patient.

Summary

Injuries to peripheral branches (IAN, LN, LBN) of the trigeminal nerve during the removal of M3s are known and accepted risks in oral and maxillofacial surgery practice. These risks might be reduced by modifications of evaluation or surgical techniques, depending on the surgeon's judgment in individual patients. If a nerve injury does occur, prompt recognition, subjective and objective evaluation, and development of a treatment plan, if the sensory deficit fails to resolve in a reasonable period and is unacceptable to the patient, give the patient the best chance of achieving improvement or recovery of sensory function in the distribution of the injured nerve. Microneurosurgery may produce return of useful sensory function or complete sensory recovery, if done in a timely fashion by an experienced microsurgeon, in greater than 80% of patients who sustain nerve injuries during the removal of M3s.

Further readings

Assael LA. Indications for elective therapeutic third molar removal: the evidence is in [editorial]. J Oral Maxillofac Surg 2005; 63:1691.

Bagheri SC, Meyer RA. Lingual nerve injury. In: Bagheri SC, JO C, editors. Clinical review of oral and maxillofacial surgery. St Louis (MO): Mosby Elsevier; 2008. p. 99–102.

Bagheri SC, Meyer RA, Ali Khan H, et al. Retrospective review of microsurgical repair of 222 lingual nerve injuries. J Oral Maxillofac Surg 2010;68:715.

Bagheri SC, Meyer RA, Cho S, et al. A retrospective review of microsurgical repair of 186 inferior alveolar nerve injuries. J Oral Maxillofac Surg 2010;68(Suppl 1):27.

Bagheri SC, Meyer RA, Etezadi H, et al. A retrospective review of microsurgical repair of long buccal nerve injuries. J Oral Maxillofac Surg 2010;68(Suppl 1):85.

Birch R, Bonney G, Wynn Parry CB. Surgical disorders of the peripheral nerves. Philadelphia: WB Saunders; 1999. p. 235–43, 405–14.

Dolanmaz D, Yildirim G, Isik K, et al. A preferable technique for protecting the inferior alveolar nerve: coronectomy. J Oral Maxillofac Surg 2009;67:1234.

Freedman GL. Intentional partial odontectomy: review of cases. J Oral Maxillofac Surg 1997;55:524.

Gomes AC, Vasconcelos BC, Silva ED, et al. Lingual nerve damage after mandibular third molar surgery: a randomized clinical trial. J Oral Maxillofac Surg 2005;63:1443.

Hatano Y, Kurita K, Kuroiwa Y, et al. Clinical evaluations of coronectomy (intentional partial odontectomy) for mandibular third molars using dental computed tomography: a case-control study. J Oral Maxillofac Surg 2009;67:1806.

Kiesselbach JE, Chamberlain JG. Clinical and anatomic observations on the relationship of the lingual nerve to the mandibular third molar region. J Oral Maxillofac Surg 1984;42:565.

Merrill RG. Prevention, treatment and prognosis for nerve injury related to the difficult impaction. Dent Clin North Am 1979;23:471.

Meyer RA. Applications of microneurosurgery to the repair of trigeminal nerve injuries. Oral Maxillofac Surg Clin North Am 1992;4:405.

Meyer RA. Nerve harvesting procedures. Atlas Oral Maxillofac Surg Clin North Am 2001;9:77.

Meyer RA, Rath EM. Sensory rehabilitation after trigeminal nerve injury or repair. Oral Maxillofac Surg Clin North Am 2001;13:365.

Meyer RA, Ruggiero SL. Guidelines for diagnosis and treatment of peripheral trigeminal nerve injuries. Oral Maxillofac Surg Clin North Am 2001;13:383.

Miloro M, Halkias LE, Slone HW, et al. Assessment of the lingual nerve in the third molar region using magnetic resonance imaging. J Oral Maxillofac Surg 1997;55:134.

Morris CD, Rasmussen J, Throckmorton GS, et al. The anatomic basis for lingual nerve trauma associated with inferior alveolar block injections. J Oral Maxillofac Surg 2010;68:2833.

Nakamori K, Fujiwara K, Miyazaki A, et al. Clinical assessment of the relationship between the third molar and the inferior alveolar canal using panoramic images and computed tomography. J Oral Maxillofac Surg 2008;66:2308.

Pogrel MA, Lee JD, Muff DF. Coronectomy: a technique to protect the inferior alveolar nerve. J Oral Maxillofac Surg 2004;62:1447–53.

Robert RC, Bacchetti P, Pogrel MA. Frequency of trigeminal nerve injuries following third molar removal. J Oral Maxillofac Surg 2005;63:732.

Roman KM. Extraction of third molars: some risk management considerations. J Ga Dent Assoc 2009;29:22 GDA Action.

Rood JP. Permanent damage to inferior alveolar and lingual nerve during the removal of impacted mandibular third molars: a comparison of two methods of bone removal. Br Dent J 1992;172:108.

Sedaghatfar M, August MA, Dodson TB. Panoramic radiographic findings as predictors of inferior alveolar nerve exposure following third molar extraction. J Oral Maxillofac Surg 2005;63:3.

Susarla SM, Dodson TB. Preoperative computed tomography imaging in the management of impacted mandibular third molars. J Oral Maxillofac Surg 2007;65:83.

Walters H. Reducing lingual nerve damage in third molar surgery: a clinical audit of 1350 cases. Br Dent J 1995;178:140.

Microsurgical Techniques for Repair of the Inferior Alveolar and Lingual Nerves

Vincent B. Ziccardi, DDS, MD

Department of Oral and Maxillofacial Surgery, New Jersey Dental School, University of Medicine and Dentistry of New Jersey, 110 Bergen Street, Room B-854, Newark, NJ 07103-2400, USA

The trigeminal nerve and its peripheral branches are susceptible to injury from maxillofacial trauma and iatrogenic causes in the practice of dentistry and medicine. These injuries can be significant for patients due to their effects on speech, mastication, food and liquid incompetence, and social interactions. Many of these sensory disturbances often undergo spontaneous recovery; however, some may be permanent with varying outcomes ranging from mild hypoesthesia to complete paresthesia. Some patients can also develop untoward outcomes such as neuropathic responses, leading to chronic pain syndromes in addition to their sensory disturbances.

The face and perioral region have one of the highest densities of peripheral nerve innervation in the body, which is why it is difficult for patients to tolerate neurologic disturbances in this region as compared with other areas. Pain, temperature, and proprioception are transmitted centrally via the lingual, mental, inferior alveolar, infraorbital, and supraorbital nerves. Each sensation is transmitted by different types of sensory receptors and nerve fibers with differing susceptibilities to injury and recovery. Each of these sensory modalities must be tested and monitored through serial examinations for spontaneous recovery in patients with peripheral trigeminal nerve injuries. The goal of trigeminal microsurgery is to create an environment in which those nerves not demonstrating spontaneous recovery are given the opportunity for regeneration and prevention of the development of neuropathies. This article reviews the indications and microsurgical techniques for repair of lingual and inferior alveolar nerve branch injuries.

Related surgical anatomy

Inferior Alveolar Nerve

The inferior alveolar nerve is the largest of the 3 branches of the mandibular division of the trigeminal nerve, which passes downward along with the inferior alveolar artery of the internal maxillary artery. The inferior alveolar nerve descends medial to the lateral pterygoid muscle and between the medial pterygoid muscle and the ramus of the mandible to enter the mandibular foramen of the mandible. The mandibular foramen is identified by an elevation called the lingula on the medial aspect of the ramus and the antelingula on the lateral surface of the ramus. In the posterior mandible, the inferior alveolar nerve is generally closer to the lingual cortical plate. The path of the inferior alveolar nerve is hyperbolic when viewed in both the sagittal and axial views from the mandibular foramen to the mental foramen. In the sagittal plane, the inferior alveolar nerve begins approximately 10 mm below the sigmoid notch and reaches its lowest point at the second premolar/molar region and then ascends superiorly to exit at the mental foramina. The inferior alveolar nerve becomes the mental nerve after it exits the mental foramen. As the inferior alveolar nerve approaches the mental foramen, it will often loop forward and then back before exiting the foramen. For this reason, the

E-mail address: ziccarvb@umdnj.edu

mental branch may be injured when surgical procedures are performed anterior to the foramen, even when the mental nerve is visualized intact outside of the mandible proper. The close approximation of the mental foramen to the dental apices accounts for the potential injuries associated with chemical, mechanical, or thermal endodontic treatment and periapical infections.

Lingual Nerve

As the lingual nerve enters the oral cavity, it travels medial to the mandibular ramus for about 3 cm. In the third molar region, the lingual nerve may be intimately associated with the third molar and/or the alveolar bone, protected by periosteum or within the soft tissues of the retromolar region. While traversing the retromandibular region, the lingual nerve can potentially cross the internal oblique ridge with only a layer of oral mucosa covering and protecting the nerve. The ultimate position of the lingual nerve at the third molar region depends on the flare of the ramus, superior position of the nerve in relation to the alveolar bone, and the third molar horizontal and vertical orientation. After looping around the submandibular duct, the lingual nerve then passes upward onto the genioglossus muscle as it enters the substance of the tongue. The lingual nerve provides several small branches that course into the mucosal lining of the medial mandible supplying the attached and unattached lingual gingival tissue up to the mandibular incisors. Injuries of the anterior tongue that are deep may also induce injury, with resulting neurosensory alterations of the tongue distal to the site of injury. In contrast to the inferior alveolar nerve, which is contained within the mandibular bone, the lingual nerve is more vulnerable to injury because of the variation of its anatomic position.

Indications for trigeminal nerve microsurgery

Indications for trigeminal nerve microsurgery include: (1) observed nerve transection, (2) no improvement in sensation for greater than 3 months, (3) development of pain due to nerve entrapment or neuroma formation, (4) presence of foreign body, (5) progressively worsening hypoesthesia or dysesthesia, and (6) hypoesthesia that is intolerable to the patient. Contraindications for trigeminal microsurgery may include: (1) development of central neuropathic pain, (2) clinical evidence of improving sensory function, (3) level of hypoesthesia that is acceptable to the patient, (4) severely medically compromised patient unable to tolerate general anesthesia for microsurgery, and (5) excessive time elapsed since the initial injury.

Nerve repairs are categorized as primary, delayed primary, and secondary depending on their timing. Primary nerve repairs are performed at the time of injury during an observed injury where the repair is immediately undertaken. If the primary surgeon is not skilled in trigeminal microsurgery, these patients may be sent to a microsurgeon who could perform the repair within a few weeks as a delayed primary repair. Unobserved injuries are the most common type of trigeminal nerve branch injury, which present to the surgeon after surgery has been completed during the postoperative period. Patients with these injuries should undergo serial neurosensory examinations to determine if trigeminal nerve microsurgery is indicated.

General principles of trigeminal nerve microsurgery

Microsurgery is performed in the operating room under general anesthesia with complete muscle relaxation. The operating room table can be turned 90° relative to the anesthesiologist to allow for placement of the surgical microscope if used; however, some surgeons prefer to use surgical loupes. An operating microscope with multiple heads is preferred by the author to allow the surgeon and assistant simultaneous views of the surgical field. Instrumentation minimally consists of micro forceps, scissors, needle holders, and nerve hooks (Figs. 1 and 2). A beaver blade is useful for the preparation of nerve ends for neurorrhaphy. Basic surgical principles for trigeminal nerve microsurgery include exposure, hemostasis, visualization, removal of scar tissue or foreign bodies, nerve preparation, and anastomosis if indicated, without tension. Residual clotted blood in proximity to a nerve repair may increase the amount of connective tissue proliferation, leading to further scarring and compression-induced ischemia potentiating demyelination, hence the importance of maintaining

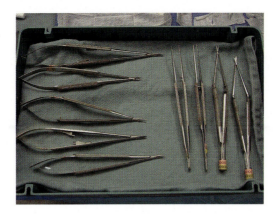

Fig. 1. Instrument tray for microsurgery.

a hemostatic surgical field. Hemostasis may be assisted through elevated head position, hypotensive general anesthesia, local anesthetic with vasoconstrictor, hemostatic agents, and bipolar electrocoagulation to minimize potential secondary injury.

Transoral approaches are commonly used for trigeminal microneurosurgery. Exposure of the inferior alveolar nerve can be accomplished after decorticating the lateral cortex through a vestibular incision with skeletonization of the mental nerve branches (Figs. 3–10). Alternatively, an extraoral submandibular incision may be indicated for those cases in which the area of injury is not easily accessible by an intraoral approach, due to restricted oral opening, local anatomy, or surgeon's preference. Regardless of which technique used to access the mandibular bone, subsequent access to the nerve is achieved through lateral decortication.

The lingual nerve is approached intraorally through either a paralingual or lingual gingival sulcus incision (Figs. 11–22). The paralingual mucosal incision is made along the floor of the mouth parallel to the lingual plate, with dissection completed using blunt and sharp dissection to expose the nerve. Advantages of this approach include a smaller incision with direct visualization; however, transected nerve ends may retract from the field on exposure. The lingual gingival sulcus incision requires a lateral release along the external oblique ridge for complete flap mobilization, and is extended along the lingual sulcus of the teeth to approximately the canine region. Once the flap is elevated in a subperiosteal plane and retracted, the nerve may be visualized from below through the overlying periosteum and bluntly dissected from the flap. This technique requires a larger incision than the paralingual incision; however, the proximal and distal nerve ends will not retract during surgical dissection.

External neurolysis is the surgical procedure used to release the nerve from its tissue bed and remove any restrictions that can lead to conduction blockade or prevent recovery. Injury to soft tissues surrounding a nerve such as the lingual nerve can induce scar tissue and create a compressive neuropathic injury. The dissection of scar tissue from an intact nerve may potentiate the recovery of

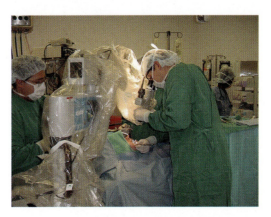

Fig. 2. Multi-head operating microscope.

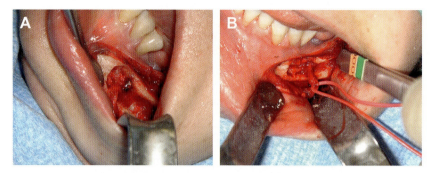

Fig. 3. (*A*) Complete inferior alveolar nerve injury related to implant placement. (*B*) Repair of inferior alveolar nerve after sacrifice of incisive branch.

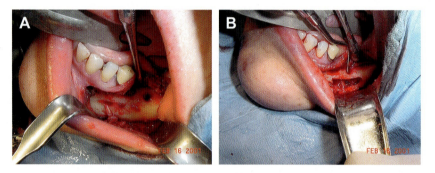

Fig. 4. (*A*) Exposure of mandible and isolation of mental nerve branches in preparation for decortication to expose the inferior alveolar nerve. (*B*) Decortication of inferior alveolar nerve with probe inserted into prior implant osteotomy site.

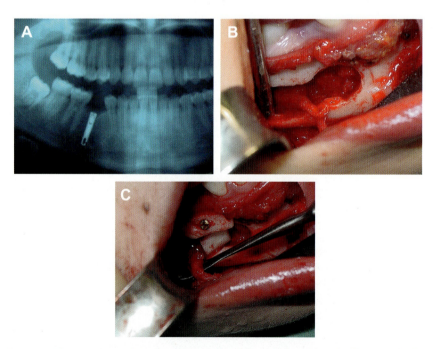

Fig. 5. (*A*) Panoramic film depicting implant placement over the shadow of the inferior alveolar nerve. Implant was subsequently removed by referring surgeon before microsurgery. (*B*) Exposure of the inferior alveolar nerve depicting complete injury. (*C*) Microrepair of the inferior alveolar nerve and bone graft to defect.

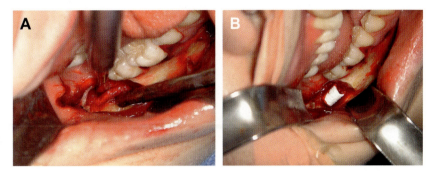

Fig. 6. (*A*) Exposure of the inferior alveolar nerve after decortication of the third molar socket. (*B*) Entubulization using collagen tubule of the inferior alveolar nerve after microrepair.

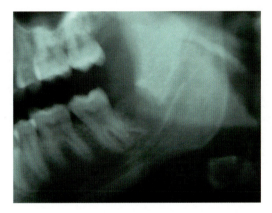

Fig. 7. Panoramic image of patient with continuity of the third molar socket with the outline of the inferior alveolar nerve. The patient sustained injury related to the removal of the symptomatic tooth.

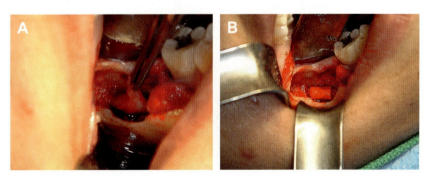

Fig. 8. (*A*) Lateral exophytic neuroma related to partial injury of the inferior alveolar nerve in the third molar socket. (*B*) Collagen tubule entubulization of the inferior alveolar nerve after microrepair.

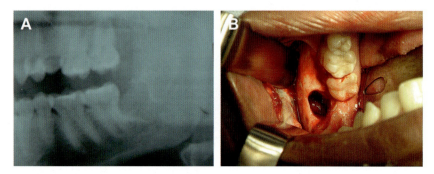

Fig. 9. (*A*) Panoramic film depicting outline of the third molar socket over the inferior alveolar nerve canal. The patient sustained and observed injury, and was immediately referred by the treating surgeon. (*B*) Exposure of the inferior alveolar nerve as visualized through third molar socket.

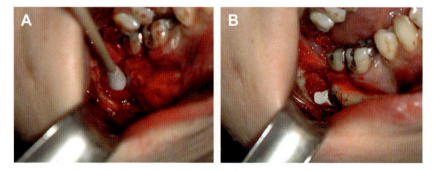

Fig. 10. (*A*) Inferior alveolar nerve after decompression as viewed through the osteotomy site. (*B*) Collagen entubulization of the inferior alveolar nerve after microrepair.

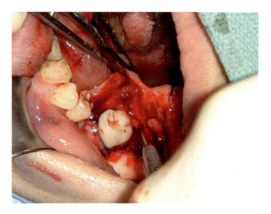

Fig. 11. Exposure of lingual nerve depicting complete injury using a crevicular incision design. Note the high position of the lingual nerve relative to the alveolar crest.

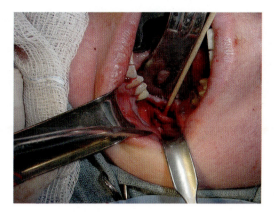

Fig. 12. Lingual nerve after decompression of the soft tissue structures.

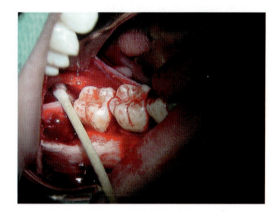

Fig. 13. Exposure of lingual nerve after decompression. The position of the nerve was over the retromolar tissues when the flap was repositioned.

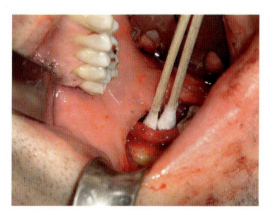

Fig. 14. Lingual nerve exposure after decompression with posterior dissection.

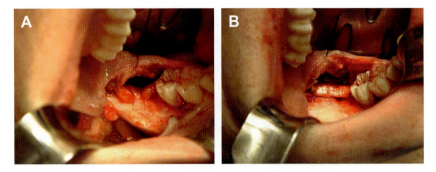

Fig. 15. (*A*) Lingual nerve with complete injury. Note the passive position of the nerve along the retromolar region. (*B*) Collagen entubulization of the lingual nerve after microrepair.

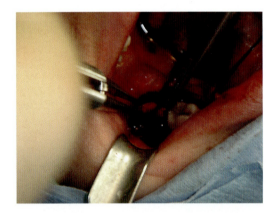

Fig. 16. Lingual nerve injury with significant scar tissue associated with stumps.

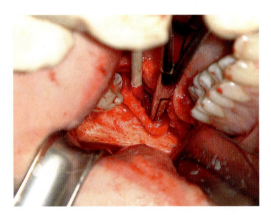

Fig. 17. Lingual nerve exposure depicting superior orientation of the nerve after repair.

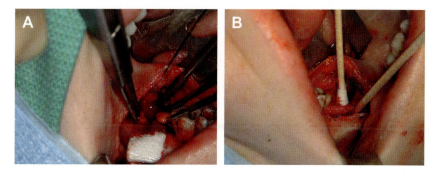

Fig. 18. (*A*) Complete injury of the lingual nerve prior to preparation for neurorrhaphy. (*B*) Microrepair of lingual nerve prior to entubulization.

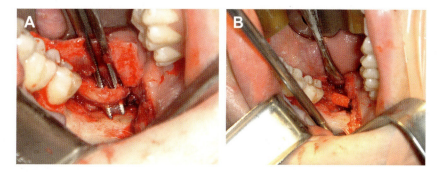

Fig. 19. (*A*) Lingual nerve exposure depicting during dissection. (*B*) Entubulization of the lingual nerve. Note the deformity of the bone in the lingual crest proximal to the injury site.

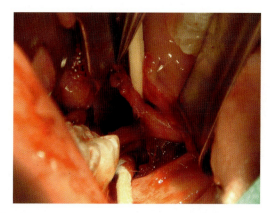

Fig. 20. Partial injury of the lingual nerve as progressing from proximal to distal.

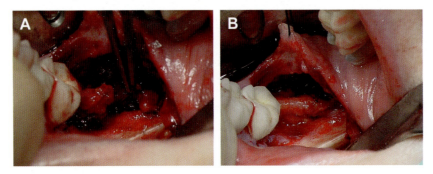

Fig. 21. (A) Complete lingual nerve injury with significant scar tissue evident on proximal and distal stumps. (B) Microrepair of lingual nerve prior to entubulization.

sensation. External neurolysis is usually performed under some magnification to grossly assess the nerve and to isolate any pathologic tissues. For patients with moderate sensory disturbances, external neurolysis may be the only surgical procedure indicated. Once the external neurolysis is completed, the nerve can be examined under magnification, and clinical findings will dictate the need for any additional procedures such as removal of foreign bodies including endodontic filling material, tooth fragments, or dental implants.

Internal neurolysis may be indicated when there is evidence of nerve fibrosis or visible regions of nerve compression. The nerve may appear narrow or enlarged depending on the mechanism and type of injury. This procedure requires opening of the epineurium to examine the internal structure of the nerve. Because the trigeminal nerve has a sparse amount of epineurium, any manipulation could potentially lead to further scar formation, hence the need for a delicate surgical technique. A longitudinal incision is made through the epineurium using a beaver blade to expose the internal structures in a procedure referred to as an epifascicular epineurotomy. With release of the epineural fibrosis the nerve may expand, indicating a successful internal neurolysis procedure. If this is ineffective, a circumferential portion of the epineurium may be removed in a procedure called epifascicular epineurectomy. If there is no expansion and fibrosis is observed, the affected nonviable segment can be excised and the nerve prepared for primary neurorrhaphy. The epineurectomy procedure is rarely indicated because of the potential for further nerve injury through the surgical manipulation itself.

Excision of neuromas is performed to prepare the nerve for reanastomosis by removing nonviable tissues in order to reestablish continuity. This procedure may be performed in cases of complete transection injuries or partial injuries in which there is an exophytic type of neuroma. After excision of the neuroma-like tissue, the resulting stumps are examined under magnification to ascertain whether normal tissue is present as determined by the presence of herniated intrafascicular tissues. The goal is to allow the suturing of the 2 nerve ends together without tension in a process called primary neurorrhaphy. The 2 nerve stumps are approximated using 7-0 to 8-0 nonreactive epineural sutures. Three to 4 sutures are optimally placed to allow for nerve healing. Nerve repair may be

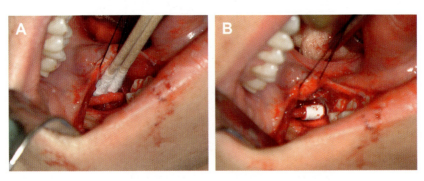

Fig. 22. (A) Decompression of the lingual nerve localized above the lingual crest. (B) Entubulization of the lingual nerve prior to wound closure.

performed at the level of the epineurium or perineurium. For purposes of peripheral trigeminal nerve repairs, an epineural suturing technique is generally performed. A suture of a nonreactive material such as nylon, smaller than 7-0 diameter, is usually selected to minimize proliferation of scar tissue. Regardless of the suture technique selected, tension across the nerve repair is minimized to prevent cell death, fibrosis, and failure of nerve regeneration. It is the preference of the author to wrap the nerve on completion with a resorbable membrane such as Neuragen (Integra Life Sciences Corporation, Plainsboro, NJ, USA) or Axoguard Nerve Protector (AxoGen Inc, Alachua, FL, USA) to protect the surgical site and potentially minimize additional scarring in the region. These materials may also provide a "seal," which ensures that growth factors released during nerve regeneration remain locally within the conduits themselves.

Outcomes of trigeminal nerve microsurgery

The clinical literature on the outcome of trigeminal nerve microsurgery is limited mostly to studies involving case reports and case series. Dodson and Kaban completed an evidence-based medicine study evaluating outcomes to develop treatment guidelines derived from the available clinical literature. Their recommendations for the management of trigeminal nerve injuries are as follows:

1. Tension-free primary repair provides the optimal result
2. If direct primary repair is not possible, autogenous nerve grafts should be used
3. When direct primary repair is not possible, autogenous nerve grafts or hollow conduits used for entubulization of nerve gaps are equally successful for delayed reconstruction of gaps 3 cm or smaller.

Pogrel reviewed patients referred over a 5-year period with the diagnosis of lingual and inferior alveolar nerve injuries. In this study of 880 consecutive patients, 96 patients met the criteria for microsurgery and 51 patients underwent a surgical procedure. No differences were observed in the results based on gender, with slightly better success in the inferior alveolar nerve group than in the lingual nerve group. Early repairs defined as those completed before 10 weeks after injury appeared to do better than later repairs. It was concluded that in select cases, trigeminal nerve microsurgery could provide a reasonable outcome, with improved sensation for inferior alveolar and lingual nerve injuries. It can be concluded that patients under proper selection criteria do benefit from trigeminal nerve microsurgery.

Further readings

Behnia H, Kheradvar A, Shabrohbi M. An anatomic study of the lingual nerve in the third molar region. J Oral Maxillofac Surg 2000;58:649–51.

Dodson TB, Kaban LB. Recommendations for management of trigeminal nerve defects based on a critical appraisal of the literature. J Oral Maxillofac Surg 1997;55:1380–6.

Donoff RB. Surgical management of inferior alveolar nerve injuries part I: the case for early repair. J Oral Maxillofac Surg 1995;53:1327.

Gulicher D, Gerlach KL. Sensory impairment of the lingual and inferior alveolar nerves following removal of impacted mandibular third molars. Int J Oral Maxillofac Surg 2001;30:306–12.

Joshi A, Rood JP. External neurolysis of the lingual nerve. Int J Oral Maxillofac Surg 2002;31:40–3.

Meyer RA. Applications of microneurosurgery to the repair of trigeminal nerve injuries. Oral Maxillofac Surg Clin North Am 1992;4:405–16.

Miloro M, Halkias LE, Slone HW, et al. Assessment of the lingual nerve in the third molar region using magnetic resonance imaging. J Oral Maxillofac Surg 1997;55:134–7.

Pogrel MA. The results of microneurosurgery of the inferior alveolar and lingual nerve. J Oral Maxillofac Surg 2002;60:485–9.

Robinson PP, Loescher AR, Smith KG. A prospective, quantitative study on the clinical outcome of lingual nerve repair. Br J Oral Maxillofac Surg 2000;38:255.

Robinson PP, Loescher AR, Yates JM, et al. Current management of damage to the inferior alveolar and lingual nerves as a result of removal of third molars. Br J Oral Maxillofac Surg 2004;42:285.

Rutner TW, Ziccardi VB, Janal MN. Long-term outcome assessment for lingual nerve microsurgery. J Oral Maxillofac Surg 2005;63:1145.

Strauss ER, Ziccardi VB, Janal MN. Outcome assessment of inferior alveolar nerve microsurgery: a retrospective review. J Oral Maxillofac Surg 2006;64:1767.

Susarla SM, Kaban LB, Donoff RB, et al. Functional sensory recovery after trigeminal nerve repair. J Oral Maxillofac Surg 2007;65:60.

Susarla SM, Kaban KB, Donoff RB, et al. Does early repair of lingual nerve injuries improve functional sensory recovery? J Oral Maxillofac Surg 2007;65:1070.

Ziccardi VB, Steinberg MJ. Timing of trigeminal nerve microsurgery: a review of the literature. J Oral Maxillofac Surg 2007;65:1341.

Ziccardi VB, Zuniga JR. Traumatic injuries of the trigeminal nerve. In: Fonseca RJ, Walker RV, Betts NJ, et al, editors. Oral and maxillofacial trauma, vol. 2. St Louis (MO): Elsevier Saunders; 2005. p. 877–914.

Ziccardi VB, Assael LA. Mechanisms of trigeminal nerve injuries. Atlas Oral Maxillofac Surg Clin North Am 2001;9:1–11.

Zuniga JR, LaBanc JP. Advances in microsurgical nerve repair. J Oral Maxillofac Surg 1993;51(Suppl 1):62–8.

Autogenous Grafts/Allografts/Conduits for Bridging Peripheral Trigeminal Nerve Gaps

Larry M. Wolford, DMD[a,b,*], Daniel B. Rodrigues, DDS[c,d]

[a]Department of Oral and Maxillofacial Surgery, Texas A&M University Health Science Center, Baylor College of Dentistry, Dallas, TX, USA
[b]Private Practice, Baylor University Medical Center, Dallas, TX, USA
[c]Department of Oral and Maxillofacial Surgery, Baylor University Medical Center, Texas A&M University Health Science Center, Baylor College of Dentistry, Dallas, TX, USA
[d]Private Practice, Salvador, Brazil

Some nerve injuries require repair in order to regain sensory or motor function. Although this article focuses primarily on trigeminal nerve (TN) injuries and repairs, the facts presented may apply to any peripheral nerve repair. The primary indications for nerve repair or grafting are (1) an injury or continuity defect in a nerve, because of trauma, pathologic condition, surgery, or disease, that cannot regain normal function without surgical intervention and (2) loss of normal neurologic function, resulting in anesthesia, paresthesia, dysesthesia, or paralysis, that cannot be corrected by nonsurgical treatment. In some nerve injuries (eg, neurapraxia), the nerve regains sensory or motor function unless irreversible compression, neuroma (axonotmesis), or transection (neurotmesis) occurs. In more severe injuries, there may be a significant loss of nerve substance (continuity defect) or a section of nerve may need to be removed to expose normal nerve tissue in preparation for nerve repair. Thus, nerve repair and nerve grafting procedures may be required to provide continuity between the proximal and distal portions of the nerve.

The 3 major branches of the TN that can be injured are the inferior alveolar nerve (IAN), lingual nerve (LN), and infraorbital nerve (ION). The most common types of injury to the IAN and LN are iatrogenic, related to the removal of impacted teeth (Fig. 1), orthognathic surgery (Fig. 2), periodontic surgery, endodontic surgery (Fig. 3), dental implants (Fig. 4), curettage of intrabony lesions, partial or total resection of the mandible or tongue in tumor removal, other surgical procedures, as well as trauma. Injuries to the ION are more commonly caused by trauma to the middle third of the face (Fig. 5A), partial or total maxillectomy and orbital exoneration during resection of benign or malignant tumors, or inadvertent nerve injury during maxillary and midface osteotomy. Nerve injuries that are more difficult to manage include severe stretch injuries and chemical injuries such as those that occur when alcohol, steroids, or other caustic agents are injected into or around nerves (see Fig. 3). The nature and extent of the nerve abnormality will influence the type and quality of repair.

Considerations for direct nerve repair

When surgical repair is required for a transected nerve or a nerve injury requiring excision, the best results, when conditions permit, are achieved with a direct nerve repair, without grafting. There are basically 3 types of nerve repair.

Perineural repair involves repairing the individual fascicles and placing sutures through the perineurium. Complications of this technique include trauma to the nerve in dissecting out each fascicle and fibrosis that develops because of the dissections and numerous sutures placed.

The authors have no competition-of-interest and no funding support.
* Corresponding author. 3409 Worth Street, Suite 400, Dallas, TX 75246.
E-mail address: lwolford@swbell.net

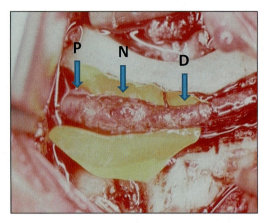

Fig. 1. A large traumatic neuroma (N) is seen 1 year after removal of the third molar. Note the significant atrophy of the distal (D) portion of the nerve and the mismatch in size compared with the proximal (P) portion of the nerve.

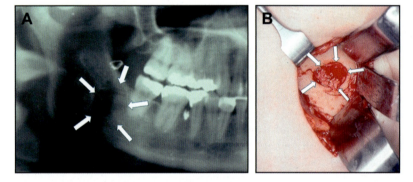

Fig. 2. (*A*) A posterior-directed lateral osteotomy for a sagittal split injured the IAN causing a large neuroma (*arrows*) that created a bone defect in the buccal cortical plate. (*B*) The neuroma (*arrows*) is observed through an extraoral approach.

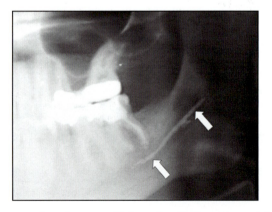

Fig. 3. A root canal procedure was performed on a mandibular molar with Sargenti paste injected into the root canals with extravasation into the IAN canal. This caustic material causes severe nerve damage (*arrows*) that adversely affects the nerve beyond the extent of the material.

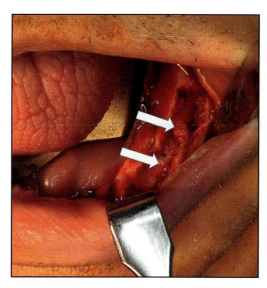

Fig. 4. This nerve injury resulted from the placement of a dental implant that crushed the IAN. The injured nerve is between the arrows. Note the atrophy of the distal nerve segment.

Group funicular repair involves repairing grouped fascicles with sutures placed through the intraneural epineurium, aligning groups of fascicles. The TN branches have nongrouped fascicles, so this technique is not applicable.

Epineural repair involves aligning the nerve ends and placing sutures through the epineurium only. Because the TN branches are polyfascicular (multiple different-sized fascicles) and nongrouped, the epineural technique is the most logical choice of repair method (Fig. 6).

Considerations for autogenous nerve grafts

When continuity defects are present in the injured nerve or created in preparation of nerve repair, a nerve graft procedure may be indicated. An additional indication includes nerve sharing in which the proximal end of a nerve is severely damaged and nonfunctional but the distal aspect can be salvaged. A portion of another nerve is isolated and a nerve graft attached and anastomosed to the distal end of the injured nerve (Fig. 7). There are various types of donor nerve grafts available. An autogenous graft is transplanted from one site to another in the same recipient, an isograft is transplanted between genetically identical or nearly identical individuals, an allograft is transplanted between genetically nonidentical individuals of the same species, and a xenograft is transplanted from the donor site of one species into the recipient site of another species.

The 2 most common autogenous donor nerves for TN repair are the sural and great auricular nerves. Selection of a donor nerve is predicated in part on the ease of harvesting and on minimizing

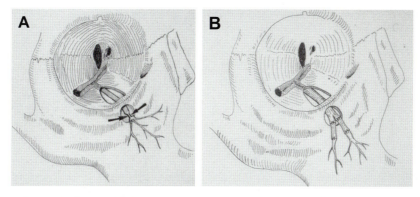

Fig. 5. (A) A crush injury to the right ION from a previous zygomaticoorbital fracture. (B) The nerve has been repaired with nerve grafts taken from the great auricular nerve.

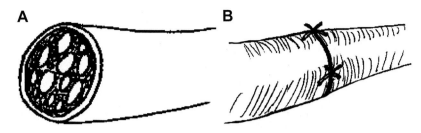

Fig. 6. (A) Because the TN branches are polyfascicular and nongrouped, (B) epineural repair is the logical choice.

post surgical symptoms associated with the donor nerve and its functional distribution. Both the sural and great auricular nerves are relatively easy to harvest but yield localized areas of sensory deficit after surgery. Other potential donor nerves include the saphenous dorsal cutaneous branch of the ulnar nerve, medial antebrachial cutaneous nerve, lateral antebrachial cutaneous nerve, superficial branches of the radial and intercostal nerves, and other branches of the cervical plexus. Several factors that are important to consider when selecting a donor nerve are addressed in the following sections.

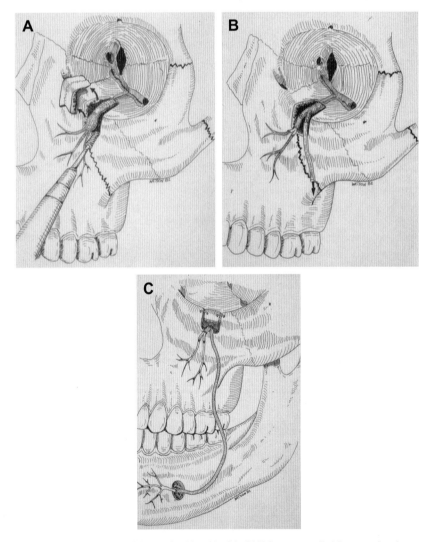

Fig. 7. (A) An injury to the ION and loss of the proximal branch of the IAN from severe facial trauma, but the mental nerve was still present. (B) The ION was divided with short sural nerve grafts used to reanastomose the distal branches of the ION and a long graft from the other part of the proximal ION, (C) to anastomose to the mental nerve. In this case, the patient did regain some sensibility to the distribution of these nerve branches.

Diameters of Donor and Host Nerves

Ideally, the diameter of the nerve graft should correlate exactly with the diameter of the proximal and distal ends of the prepared host nerve. The average diameters of the IAN, LN, sural nerve, and great auricular nerve are 2.4 mm, 3.2 mm, 2.1 mm, and 1.5 mm, respectively. For IAN grafting, the sural nerve is generally considered the best cross-sectional match because its diameter is 87% that of the IAN but only 66% that of the LN. The great auricular nerve diameter is about 63% of the IAN diameter and 47% of the LN diameter. The great auricular nerve works best if placed as a cable graft (Fig. 8), with 2 or more parallel graft strands, so that the combined diameter of the 2 strands would be adequate (125% of the IAN and 94% of the LN diameters).

Length of Nerve Graft Required

It may be difficult to obtain a graft longer than 2 to 4 cm from the great auricular nerve. Because the diameter of the great auricular nerve (Fig. 9A) is generally half the diameter of the IAN and LN, a 2-strand cable graft usually works best for diameter match (see Fig. 8). Therefore, it may be difficult to graft a defect larger than 1 to 1.5 cm if the graft is harvested unilaterally. The sural nerve is larger in diameter, and a 20 to 30 cm length can be harvested without much difficulty (see Fig. 9B). Because a longer graft will usually be necessary for nerve-sharing techniques, the sural nerve would be the autogenous donor choice (see Fig. 7A, B).

Number of Fascicles

The number and size of fascicles should correlate between the donor and host nerves. The IAN usually has 18 to 21 fascicles in the third molar area (Fig. 10A), decreasing to about 12 fascicles just proximal to the mental foramen area (see Fig. 10B) [1,2]. The LN in the third molar area usually has 15 to 18 fascicles, decreasing to 9 fascicles as it enters the tongue. The sural nerve usually has 11 to 12 fascicles, which is 54% of the number of fascicles in the IAN and 69% of the number in the LN. The great auricular nerve usually has 8 to 9 fascicles, which is significantly less than the number in the IAN (44%) and LN (52%). However, if a cable graft with 2 parallel nerve graft strands is used (see Fig. 8), the combined number of fascicles correlates more closely with those of the IAN (87%) and LN (104%). Sometimes, the great auricular nerve is even smaller, and the transverse cervical nerve may be considered. If the nerve graft is significantly smaller in diameter than the proximal host nerve stump, fascicles are lost and a neuroma may form. If the graft is too large at the distal host nerve stump, some of the regenerating nerve fascicles in the graft will be lost. If the distal portion of the graft is smaller than the distal portion of the host nerve, several fascicles in the distal portion of the host nerve will not regenerate.

Fascicular Pattern

The IAN and LN have polyfascicular patterns; the fascicular size ranges from small to large diameter, but without fascicular grouping. The sural nerve has an oligofascicular (uniform size) pattern, but with small-diameter fascicles. The great auricular nerve is a polyfascicular nerve with grouping, a pattern that more closely approximates the fascicular pattern of the IAN and LN than that of the sural nerve. The axons in the sural nerve are much smaller and fewer than those in the IAN and LN, creating another significant mismatch.

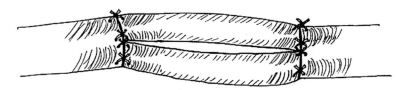

Fig. 8. The cable grafting technique may be indicated to improve the match of graft to host nerve in the cross-sectional diameter, number of fascicles, and fascicular pattern.

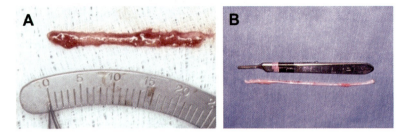

Fig. 9. (A) The great auricular nerve provides a shorter length of graft and the diameter is significantly smaller than that of the TN branches. (B) A significantly longer graft can be harvested from the sural nerve and it has a larger diameter than the great auricular nerve.

Cross-sectional Shape and Area

The IAN and LN are round, whereas the sural nerve is basically flat. The great auricular nerve is round to oval. Therefore, the great auricular nerve more closely resembles the IAN and LN than the sural nerve. The approximate total cross-sectional area of the IAN is 4.6 mm^2; the LN, 5.2 mm^2; the sural nerve, 3.5 mm^2; and the great auricular nerve, 1.8 mm^2. There is no significant difference in the fascicular and total nerve areas among the IAN, LN, and great auricular nerve. The sural nerve has significantly smaller axonal size and number of axons per unit area (50% less) than the others.

Patient Preference

Harvesting the sural nerve results in numbness of the heel and lateral aspect of the foot (Fig. 11). Harvesting the great auricular nerve results in numbness to the ear, lateral part of the neck, and the skin overlying the posterior aspect of the mandible (Fig. 12). An additional risk at the donor area is the development of a painful neuroma that may require additional treatment. Patients may prefer that their numbness and/or potential complications be in the foot or in the head and neck area.

Factors affecting nerve graft success

The success and ultimate outcome of a nerve repair or grafting procedure are based on several factors; the more favorable the factors, the better and more predictable the outcome.

Time Since the Injury

Peripheral nerve injuries requiring surgical intervention will have better results the earlier the nerve is repaired after injury. Therefore, repairs with or without grafting done immediately after the injury yield better results, with progressively worsening results if done 3, 6, 9, or 12 months or longer after the injury. Wietholter and colleagues [3] reported best results for IAN and LN repairs if reconstruction was done within 3 weeks of the injury. Early repair circumvents major problems

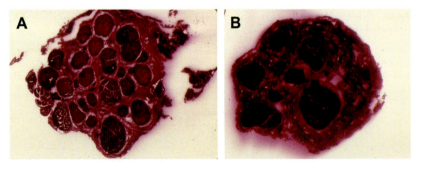

Fig. 10. (A) This cross-sectional histologic view of the IAN at the third molar area shows the polyfascicular pattern. (B) Just proximal to the mental foramen, the number of fascicles in the IAN significantly decreases.

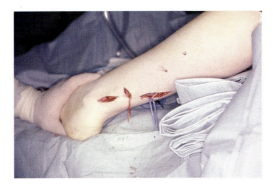

Fig. 11. The sural nerve is harvested through multiple small incisions in the lower part of the leg.

encountered with elapsed time, such as wallerian degeneration, atrophy, and fibrosis in the distal portion of the nerve (see Fig. 1). Atrophy creates a significant size match discrepancy between the nerve graft and either or both stumps. The time factor reflects the rate and extent of degeneration and atrophy of the distal fascicles before nerve repair. However, if the injury is primarily a traumatic neuroma without atrophy or degenerative neurologic changes in the distal portion of the nerve, the time factor may not be as important; that is, whether the repair is done at 3 weeks or 2 years may not make a difference in the functional outcome.

Type and Extent of Injury

The more localized and confined the injury, the lesser the trauma to the nerve, and the shorter the required nerve graft (or possibility of repair without grafting), the better the outcome. Stretch injuries or injuries caused by injection of alcohol, steroids, or other caustic chemicals into or adjacent to a nerve (see Fig. 3) can cause significant irreversible damage to the nerve, which can extend

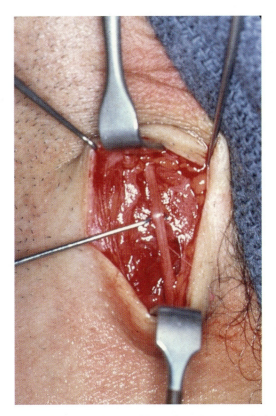

Fig. 12. The great auricular nerve is harvested from the neck through a horizontal incision.

proximally into the ganglion and cell bodies, beyond a surgically accessible area, thus rendering peripheral nerve repair ineffective.

Vascularity in Host Bed

For a nerve graft to be successful, it must be revascularized quickly. Therefore, having the graft and the areas of anastomosis exposed to adjacent healthy soft tissues will help in this regard. Placing the graft inside a bony canal or in an area of significant scar tissue will predictably have poorer results because of delayed revascularization of the graft.

Orientation of Nerve Graft Placement

A nerve graft should be placed so that it is oriented in the same functional direction from which it was harvested. That is, the proximal end of the nerve graft should approximate the proximal end of the host nerve and the distal end of the graft should anastomose with the distal end of the host nerve. Axonoplasmic flow should be maintained in the same direction. Therefore, when a nerve graft is harvested, the orientation should be carefully noted.

Length of Nerve Graft Required

The shorter the nerve graft required, the better the result. The longer the nerve graft, the less predictable the result. This difference in result is due in part to the amount of time it takes for regeneration to occur across each anastomosis area (7–14 days) and along the length of the nerve (0.2–3 mm/d). The longer the nerve graft, the more is the time required for regeneration to reach the distal anastomosis of the graft, increasing the risk of atrophy and fibrous ingrowth into the distal anastomosis area, resulting in a poorer outcome (see Fig. 7).

Quality and Type of Repair

Quality of repair is particularly sensitive to the surgeon's skill and experience. Obviously, the highest quality repairs yield the best results. A high-quality repair includes atraumatic management of the proximal and distal ends of the host and graft nerves. The TN branches are polyfascicular and have no grouping, so epineural repair is the most logical and appropriate technique (see Fig. 6). Depending on the situation, 8-0 to 10-0 monofilament nylon suture can be used for the repairs. Minimizing the number of sutures (3–6 is optimal) is helpful as long as the approximation of the graft to the nerve stumps is accurate. It is important to try to suture only the epineurium and not pass the needle and suture through the fascicles because this can create more damage and scarring, yielding a poorer result.

Tension on Repaired Nerve

The nerve should be repaired or grafted with no tension on the nerve segments and areas of anastomosis (Fig. 13). Excessive tension can cause breakdown at the area of anastomosis, resulting in a poor outcome. The host nerve should be prepared before harvesting the graft so that graft length can be determined as accurately as possible. The cut host nerve will retract, yielding a larger defect. A harvested nerve graft shrinks in length by approximately 20%, and additional length may be lost in final preparation of host and nerve graft ends. Therefore, the nerve graft harvested should be at least 25% longer than the host nerve defect to compensate for these changes.

Preparation of the Host Nerve

A good result requires removal of the area of injury and assurance of healthy viable nerve at the proximal and distal stumps. Frozen sections for histologic assessment of the proximal and distal stumps may be helpful to determine when good viable nerve tissue has been reached. In the distal end, there may be degenerative changes (wallerian degeneration) involving the fascicles. However, it is important to be sure that no significant fibrosis or other obstructions remain in the distal portion of the host nerve (Fig. 14).

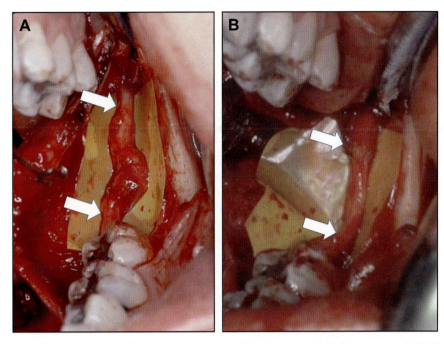

Fig. 13. (A) LN with a large neuroma (*between the arrows*) caused by of an impacted third molar removal. (B) The nerve has been repaired with a sural nerve graft (*between the arrows*) without any tension on the nerve segments.

Age of Patient and Other Health Factors

In general, young children have the best results, and elderly patients, the poorest results for nerve repair or grafting. Children have a greater ability to centrally adapt to altered nerve programming, greater regenerative capabilities, and greater healing and metabolic rates than older patients. Systemic factors that can adversely affect outcome include connective tissue and autoimmune diseases (eg, scleroderma, mixed connective tissue disease, rheumatoid diseases, systemic lupus erythematosus), diabetes, vascular and bleeding disorders, inherited or acquired neuropathies, alcoholism, and smoking. These factors must be considered when counseling patients about the risks, complications, and expected outcomes.

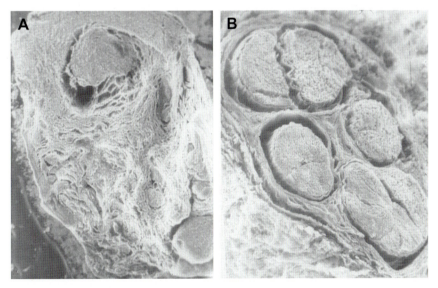

Fig. 14. (A) Frozen section of an injured proximal nerve segment shows significant fibrosis and no viable fascicles. (B) Frozen nerve section further proximal demonstrates viable nerve tissue.

Expected outcomes

Many factors influence the quality of results. If the donor nerve and other success factors are all favorable, good results can be expected. Definition of a successful and acceptable outcome varies widely among patients and surgeons. The quality of outcome for a given patient may not be predictable, but the more favorable the factors affecting success, the greater the potential for a good outcome. It must be understood that the best result may not restore function to the preinjury level. With an LN injury, return of taste sensation should not be expected.

Wietholter and colleagues [3] found better results for IAN repair with end-to-end anastomosis than with nerve grafting. The senior author, Larry M. Wolford has also had this experience. Therefore, with IAN injuries, the possibility of decortication of the mandible over the distal portion of the IAN should be evaluated and the distal portion of the IAN and mental nerve should be posteriorly repositioned to facilitate an end-to-end repair before considering a nerve graft. Hessling and colleagues [4] reported that only 40% of patients who underwent IAN reconstruction and 35% who underwent LN reconstruction had good results. They recommended reconstruction of these nerves only if the patient has pain in addition to loss of sensitivity. Zuniga [5] reported on the outcomes of nerve repair in 10 patients; both the patients and the surgeon rated the overall outcomes as mostly good, although there were differences in specific outcome ratings by surgeon and patients. Donoff and Colin [6] reported improvement in 63% of their patients who underwent LN repair (31 nerves): 77% in the anesthesia group and 42% in the pain-paresthesia group. Improvement was seen in 77% of patients who underwent IAN repair.

Less-favorable results in some studies may be related to unfavorable factors affecting outcome. Assessment of the literature indicates that LN repairs are less successful than other nerve repairs. Perhaps, difficulty in surgical access and constant mobility of the area after surgery (ie, eating, swallowing, speaking) may contribute to the lower success rate. Also, the LN is the largest branch of the trigeminal system. Most surgeons use only a single-strand graft for repair of any of the TN branches, resulting in a significant mismatch in size and fascicular characteristics, which may contribute to a less-satisfactory outcome. Use of cable grafting may improve the results for some patients.

Nerve grafting with other tissues

Alternative tissues such as veins, collagen conduits and filaments, and perineurium tubes have been used for nerve repair. Most human studies have involved vein grafts. There are no studies on using vein grafts for repair of the TN branches. Tang and colleagues [7] reported on a technique in which a vein was taken from the forearm and reversed to bridge digital nerve defects. For nerve defects larger than 2 cm, normal nerve slices were inserted inside vein conduits. Follow-up revealed excellent recovery in 2 digital nerves, good in 9, fair in 5, and poor in 2.

Chiu and Strauch [8] reported a prospective comparative clinical study evaluating direct nerve repair, nerve grafting, and vein grafting for distal sensory nerve defects smaller than 3 cm. A total of 34 nerves were repaired: 15 with a venous nerve conduit, 4 with a sural nerve graft, and 15 with direct repair. Significant symptom relief and satisfactory sensory function return were observed in all patients. Two-point discrimination measurements indicated the superiority of direct repair, followed by conventional nerve grafting and then vein grafting. However, the universally favorable patient acceptance and the return of measurable 2-point discrimination indicated the effectiveness of autogenous vein grafts as nerve conduits when selectively applied to bridge a small nerve gap (<3 cm) on nonessential peripheral sensory nerves.

Walton and colleagues [9] reported a retrospective study on the use of autogenous vein grafts in 22 digital nerve repairs. The 2-point discrimination averaged 4.6 mm for 11 acute digital nerve repairs using vein conduits 1 to 3 cm in length. Delayed digital nerve repair with vein conduits yielded poor results. Comparing end-to-end digital nerve repairs and digital nerve grafting suggests that repair of 1- to 3-cm gaps in digital nerves with segments of autologous vein grafts seems to give results comparable to those of nerve grafting.

However, autogenous vein grafts have little mechanical resistance to kinking and collapse. Tang and colleagues [10] demonstrated that repair of digital nerves with gaps ranging from 4 to 5.8 cm using vein conduits yielded no detectable recovery of sensibility in autonomous areas of these nerves and no sign of recovery of the innervated muscles during follow-up. Reexploration revealed that the vein conduits used for repair of the median nerves were constricted by the surrounding scar tissue; axon regeneration was precluded.

Alloplastic nerve grafts

Permanent Conduit Materials

Silicone is a permanent conduit material that has been used for nerve grafting. However, long-term tubulization of a nerve produces localized compression with resultant decreased axonal conduction, although the total number of nerve fibers and axon size remain constant. Alterations in the blood-nerve barrier occur, followed by demyelination of the nerve fibers. Silicone tubes used for neural conduits must be removed to achieve a positive outcome [11]. Similar unfavorable outcomes occur when using Gore-Tex (polytetrafluorethylene) vein grafts (W. L. Gore and Associates Inc, Flagstaff, AZ, USA) as a nerve graft conduit (Fig. 15). Clinical studies indicated that the Gore-Tex tubing is not effective and therefore not recommended in the repair of continuity defects of the IAN and LN. The Gore-Tex tubing collapses after surgery, impeding nerve regeneration.

Synthetic Resorbable Conduits

Polyglycolic acid (Dexon, American Cyanamid Co, Wayne, NJ, USA) is a bioabsorbable substance that is currently used as a suture material in a mesh form to wrap internal organs injured because as a result of trauma. This substance is absorbed in the body by hydrolysis within 90 days of implantation. A bioabsorbable polyglycolic acid conduit has been developed for nerve grafting (Neurotube, Synovis Life Technologies Inc, St Paul, MN, USA) (Figs. 16 and 17). Characteristics of this tube include (1) porosity, which provides an oxygen-rich environment for the regenerating nerve, (2) flexibility, to accommodate movement of joints and associated tendon gliding, (3) corrugation, to resist the occlusive force of surrounding soft tissue, and (4) bioabsorbability, eliminating the need for removal at a subsequent operation. This corrugated tube has available internal diameters from 2.3 to 8 mm and lengths from 2 to 4 cm.

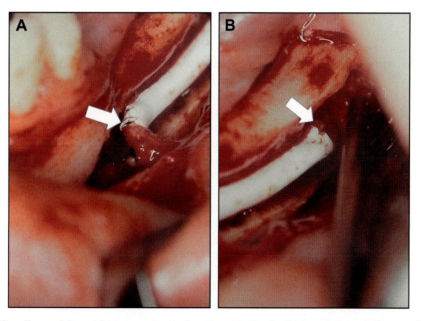

Fig. 15. (*A*) Gore-Tex conduit used for nerve reconstruction, demonstrating the distal repair (*arrow*). Because of distal nerve atrophy, the distal end of the graft has been narrowed to conform to the diameter of the distal nerve segment. This modification can be used for other conduit products. (*B*) The proximal repair is seen (*arrow*). However, Gore-Tex grafts are not recommended for the repair of TN branches.

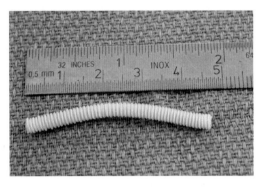

Fig. 16. Neurotube is a polyglycolic acid tube with porosity, flexibility, corrugation to resist occlusive forces, and bioabsorbability.

Weber and colleagues [12] reported a prospective study on 136 nerve repairs in the hand, divided into 2 groups: group 1 consisted of standard repair with either end-to-end anastomosis or nerve graft, and group 2 consisted of nerve repair using a Neurotube conduit (see Fig. 16). Overall, there were no statistical differences between the 2 groups. However, the 2-point discrimination was better in the Neurotube group (6.8 ± 3.8 mm) than in the direct anastomosis or nerve graft group (12.9 ± 2.4 mm). The Neurotube conduit provided superior results and eliminated donor site morbidity. Mackinnon and Dellon [13,14] reported good to excellent results in 86% of digital nerve repairs in 15 patients using Neurotube. It is recommended to fill the tube with heparinized saline. Casanas and colleagues [15] studied 17 patients with digital nerve defects ranging from 2 to 3.5 cm grafted with Neurotube with good results. Navissano and colleagues [16] reported on using Neurotube to repair facial nerve defects from 1 to 3 cm with good results in 5 of 7 patients.

Few articles have been published about Neurotube as an alloplastic material for TN repair. Crawley and Dellon [17] reported an isolated case in which a 2.0-mm diameter Neurotube conduit was used in a 51-year-old woman to repair the right IAN 16 months after injury. The Neurotube conduit was filled with autologous serum to prevent blood clot formation. At 12 months after surgery, the pressure and vibratory perception were similar to those of the contralateral lip and chin area.

Poly (DL-lactide-ϵ-caprolactone) Neurolac Nerve Guide (Polyganics Inc Groningen, The Netherlands) is another synthetic nerve conduit with a 3.5-cm length and 1.5- to 10-mm internal diameter. The tube is less flexible, tends to swell, and takes 16 to 24 months to absorb. Bertleff and colleagues [18] reported results in 54 patients with digital nerve injuries, with the controls using direct repair or nerve grafting and the experimental group treated with Neurolac conduits. Interim results showed comparable outcomes, but at longer follow-up, the Neurolac group did not show better function and had significantly more complications related to the initial stiffness of the conduits, but subsequent collapse during the absorption phase. Battiston and colleagues [19] reported on 28 digital nerve repairs with Neurolac with 93% good to excellent results.

Semipermeable collagen type 1 nerve guides have been developed (NeuraGen nerve guide, Integra LifeSciences, Plainsboro, NJ, USA). Type 1 collagen–based implants support and guide tissue regeneration in vivo, have low immunogenicity, and are biocompatible (Fig. 18). Tube lengths are 2 to 3 cm, with internal diameters from 1.5 to 7 mm, and with an absorption rate of 4 to 8 months. Ashley and colleagues [20] used NeuraGen nerve conduits in patients with brachial plexus birth injuries, with 4 of 5 patients showing good recovery at 2 years after surgery. Lohmeyer and colleagues [21] used NeuraGen grafts in hand surgery reporting 4 of 6 patients with excellent results at 1 year after surgery. There are no reports on using these conduits for IAN or LN repairs.

Nerve Cuffs

Farole and Jamal [22] described the results of using NeuraGen cuffs placed around nerve repair sites in 8 patients with 9 repairs. After primary nerve repair, a NeuraGen conduit was split longitudinally and encased around the repair site with at least 1.5 cm of margin. At 1 to 2.5 years' follow-up, 4 repairs were found to have good improvement, 4 had some improvement, and 1 had no improvement. Neuroflex NeuroMatrix (Collagen Matrix Inc, Franklin Lakes, NJ, USA) also makes a nerve cuff that is nonfriable, crimped, semipermeable tubular membrane matrix of type 1 collagen. The

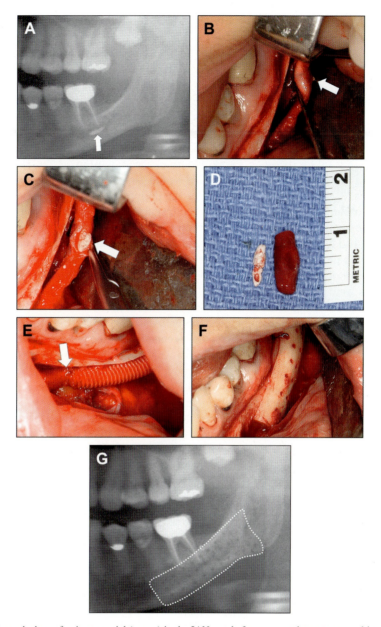

Fig. 17. (*A*) Radiograph shows foreign material (*arrow*) in the IAN canal after root canal treatment resulting in a painful dysesthesia to the distribution of the IAN. (*B*) After decortications of the mandible, the IAN has been lateralized from the mandible. The arrow points to the nerve lesion. (*C*) An incision (*arrow*) into the nerve shows a foreign body within the nerve. (*D*) The IAN lesion has been resected, and the foreign body removed. (*E*) The nerve has been repaired with 2.3-mm diameter Neurotube (*arrow*), with the distal repair observed. (*F*) The lateral cortical bone that was removed for access to the IAN is replaced in position. The holes placed in the bone are to aid in revascularization. (*G*) Radiograph shows the replaced buccal cortical bone.

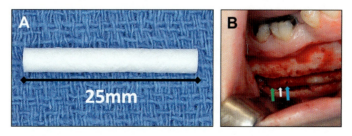

Fig. 18. (*A*) A NeuraGen nerve guide can be used for nerve repair. (*B*) The NeuroGen tube has been used to repair the IAN. The green arrow shows the proximal nerve end. The white arrow shows where the IAN inserts into the NeuroGen tube. The blue arrow points at one of the 3 sutures used to deliver the IAN within the conduit and stabilize it in place.

length is 2.5 cm, and internal diameter ranges from 2 to 6 mm with 4 to 8 months for absorption. There are no studies on application for IAN or LN.

Because these absorbable conduits disintegrate, the problems associated with permanent tubing (ie, Silastic, Gore-Tex, Dow-Corning, Midland, MO, USA), including compression and demyelination, are eliminated. The superior results achieved with nerve grafting conduits are related to the elimination of the problems associated with harvested nerve grafts, host-donor differences in diameter, mismatches in the number and pattern of fascicles and cross-sectional shape and area, as well as morbidity of the donor area. However, absorbable conduit grafting results are still affected by factors such as time since injury, type and extent of injury, vascularity, graft size match, length of nerve graft required (results are good for defects <3 cm), quality of repair, tension on the repaired nerve, preparation of the host nerve, age of patient, and other health factors.

Meek and Coert [23] recommend Neurotube as the preferred conduit for nerve repair after their extensive review of the various options. Shin and colleagues [24] performed a murine study creating 10-mm gaps in the sciatic nerve with 4 groups: group 1 had reversed autografts, group 2 had Neurolac conduits, group 3 had NeuraGen conduits, and group 4 had Neurotube conduits. Groups 1 and 2 had the best results, with no significant difference between them. Group 4 had the poorest results, partly because the diameter of the sciatic nerve was 1.5 mm and the smallest Neurotube was 2.3 mm, while the other conduits were of the appropriate size. This result further supports the importance of having diameter of the conduit coordinated to that of the host nerve.

The authors have used the Neurotube conduit for IAN and LN grafting with good preliminary results. The technique that the authors use includes preparation of the proximal and distal ends of the host nerve and of a conduit graft that is at least 1 cm longer than the size of the defect. Three to four 8-0 to 10-0 nylon sutures are passed through the tube 5 mm from the end, through the epineurium of the proximal nerve stump, and back out through the tube in a mattress fashion. After all sutures are passed, the sutures are gently pulled to deliver the proximal end of the nerve within the tube (see Figs. 16 and 17). The same procedure is performed for the distal end of the nerve. If there is a discrepancy in the sizes of host nerve end and tube diameter, the tube can be slit at the end to allow expansion or contraction to correlate to host nerve diameter. The artificial nerve conduit is then filled with a solution containing 1000 U of heparin per 100 mL of isotonic saline to help prevent blood clot formation, which could impede axonal regeneration.

Allograft nerve grafts

The cadaveric nerve allograft provides an unlimited graft source acting as viable nerve conduits without the morbidities associated with autograft reconstruction. Host motor and sensory axons grow to reach the host target via those conduits. The regenerating autologous nerves provide function, and allogenic cells support this regeneration. To ensure Schwann cell viability and minimal fibrosis, the allograft must be revascularized in an early posttransplant period.

These grafts are rapidly rejected unless appropriate immunosuppression is achieved. The toxicity associated with immunosuppression required to promote graft acceptance must be compared with the relative benefits of reinnervation before nerve allotransplantation can be safely applied in routine practice. Mackinnon and colleagues [25–27] treated 7 patients with allograft nerve transplantation, up to 37 cm in length, to the extremities with immunosuppression therapy started several days before surgery. The average time of immunosuppressive therapy was 18 months, with no posttreatment evidence of adverse reaction. One graft was rejected. The other patients at longest follow-up had light touch, hot and cold, as well as pain sensations, but no 2-point discrimination. Optimal treatment methods for nerve allograft transplantation must minimize or prevent rejection and permit nerve regeneration at the same time.

Another alternative is the use of processed allografts such as Avance (AxoGen Inc, Alachua, FL, USA), a human decellularized allograft product (Fig. 19). Processed allografts retain the scaffold of nerve tissue but are made to be nonimmunogenic and inert in the body by a variety of processing methods. Examples of processing techniques include repeated freeze-thaw cycles, exposure to radiation, extended storage in cold University of Wisconsin solution, and decellularization with detergents. Processed allografts provide a biologic substrate for nerve regeneration without the requirements of immunosuppression.

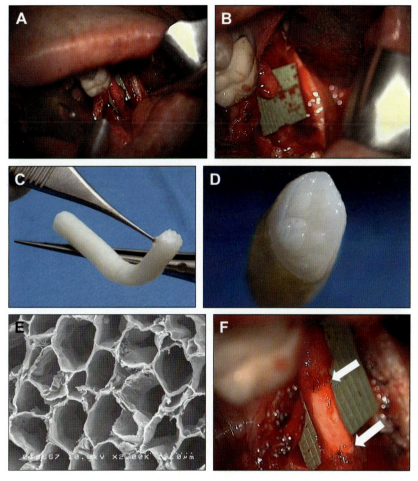

Fig. 19. (*A*) Left IAN neuroma. (*B*) The neuroma has been excised. (*C*) A 3- to 4-mm diameter × 30 mm length Avance Nerve Graft was trimmed to span the 10-mm defect. (*D*) The nerve allograft held in tweezers demonstrating handling properties. (*E*) Photomicrograph of Avance allograft at high magnification. (*F*) The IAN has been repaired with Avance decellularized cadaveric nerve. The arrows delineate the graft. (*Courtesy of* Martin Steed, DDS, Atlanta, GA [*A*, *B*, *F*].)

Whitlock and colleagues [28] used a murine model to compare isograft, NeuraGen (type I collagen conduit), and processed rat allografts comparable to Axogen's Avance. In the long sciatic nerve gap model (28 mm), the isograft was superior to processed allograft, which was in turn superior to NeuraGen conduits at 6 weeks after surgery. The investigators conclude that in the long gap model, nerve grafting alternatives fail to deliver the regenerative advantages of an isograft. However, in the short sciatic nerve gap model (14 mm) there was no significant difference between the 3 groups relative to nerve regeneration at 22 weeks. Although the use of processed decellularized cadaveric allografts looks promising for nerve injury repair, there are no studies available to determine the efficacy of using this graft system for the repair of LN or IAN injuries.

Summary

Nerve repairs and grafting techniques have been around for many years. Autogenous nerve grafts have worked reasonably well in the right circumstances but are associated with difficulties in achieving a proper donor-host match and with postsurgical sequelae at the donor site. Vein grafts seem to work almost as well as autogenous nerve grafts in digital nerve repairs that require a graft less than 3 cm in length. Currently, the most promising nerve graft materials are the polyglycolic acid tubes and processed decellularized allografts, which have shown good results without the morbidity of autogenous nerve grafts. However, more research studies using these materials for TN repairs are essential to validate the superiority of these procedures.

References

[1] Svane TJ. The fascicular characteristics of human inferior alveolar and greater auricular nerves [master's thesis]. Waco (TX): Baylor University; 1989.

[2] Svane TJ, Wolford LM, Milam SB, et al. Fascicular characteristics of the human inferior alveolar nerve. J Oral Maxillofac Surg 1986;44:431–4.

[3] Wietholter H, Riediger D, Ehrenfeld M, et al. [Results of micro-surgery of sensory peripheral branches of the mandibular nerve]. Fortschr Kiefer Gesichtschir 1990;35:128–34 [in German].

[4] Hessling KH, Reich RH, Hausamen JE, et al. [Long-term results of microsurgical nerve reconstruction in the area of the head-neck]. Fortschr Kiefer Gesichtschir 1990;35:134–8 [in German].

[5] Zuniga JR. Perceived expectation, outcome, and satisfaction of microsurgical nerve repair. J Oral Maxillofac Surg 1991;49(Suppl 1):77.

[6] Donoff RB, Colin W. Neurologic complications of oral and maxillofacial surgery. Oral Maxillofac Surg Clin North Am 1990;2:453–62.

[7] Tang JB, Gu YQ, Song YS. Repair of digital nerve defect with autogenous vein graft during flexor tendon surgery in zone 2. J Hand Surg Br 1993;18:449–53.

[8] Chiu DT, Strauch B. A prospective clinical evaluation of autogenous vein grafts used as a nerve conduit for distal sensory nerve defects of 3 cm or less. Plast Reconstr Surg 1990;86:928–34.

[9] Walton RL, Brown RE, Matory WE Jr, et al. Autogenous vein graft repair of digital nerve defects in the finger: a retrospective clinical study. Plast Reconstr Surg 1989;84:944–9.

[10] Tang JB, Shi D, Zhou H. Vein conduits for repair of nerves with a prolonged gap or in unfavorable conditions: an analysis of three failed cases. Microsurgery 1995;16:133–7.

[11] Dellon AL. Use of a silicone tube for the reconstruction of a nerve injury. J Hand Surg Br 1994;19:271–2.

[12] Weber RA, Breidenbach WC, Brown RE, et al. A randomized prospective study of polyglycolic acid conduits for digital nerve reconstruction in humans. Plast Reconstr Surg 2000;106:1036–45.

[13] Mackinnon SE, Dellon AL. Surgery of the peripheral nerve. New York: Thieme; 1988.

[14] Mackinnon SE, Dellon AL. Clinical nerve reconstruction with a bioabsorable polyglycolic acid tube. Plast Reconstr Surg 1990;85:419–24.

[15] Casanas J, Serra J, Orduna M, et al. Repair of digital sensory nerves of the hand using polyglycolic acid conduits. J Hand Surg Br 2000;25:44.

[16] Navissano M, Malan F, Carnino R, et al. Neurotube for facial nerve repair. Microsurgery 2005;25:268–71.

[17] Crawley WA, Dellon AL. Inferior alveolar nerve reconstruction with a polyglycolic acid bioabsorbable nerve conduit. Plast Reconstr Surg 1992;90:300–2.

[18] Bertleff MJ, Meek MF, Nicolai JP. A prospective clinical evaluation of biodegradable Neurolac nerve guides for sensory nerve repair in the hand. J Hand Surg Am 2005;30:513–8.

[19] Battiston B, Geuna S, Ferrero M, et al. Nerve repair by means of tubulization: literature review and personal clinical experience comparing biological and synthetic conduits for sensory nerve repair. Microsurgery 2005;25:258–67.

[20] Ashley WW, Weatherly T, Park TS. Collagen nerve guides for surgical repair of brachial plexus birth injury. J Neurosurg 2006;105:452–6.

[21] Lohmeyer J, Zimmermann S, Sommer B, et al. Bridging peripheral nerve defects by means of nerve conduits. Chirurg 2007;78:142–7.

[22] Farole A, Jamal BT. A bioabsorbable collagen nerve cuff (NeuraGen) for repair of lingual and inferior alveolar nerve injuries: a case series. J Oral Maxillofac Surg 2008;66:2058–62.

[23] Meek MF, Coert JH. US Food and Drug Administration/Conformit Europe-approved absorbable nerve conduits for clinical repair of peripheral and cranial nerves. Ann Plast Surg 2008;60:110–6.

[24] Shin RH, Friedrich PF, Crum BA, et al. Treatment of a segmental nerve defect in the rat with use of bioabsorbable synthetic nerve conduits: a comparison of commercially available conduits. J Bone Joint Surg Am 2009;91:2194–204.

[25] Mackinnon SE, Dellon AL, Hudson AR, et al. Chronic nerve compression an experimental model in the rat. Ann Plast Surg 1984;13:112–20.

[26] Mackinnon SE, Dellon AL, Hudson AR, et al. A primate model for chronic nerve compression. J Reconstr Microsurg 1985;1:185–95.

[27] Mackinnon SE, Doolabh VB, Novak CB, et al. Clinical outcome following nerve allograft transplantation. Plast Reconstr Surg 2001;107:1419–29.

[28] Whitlock EL, Tuffaha SH, Luciano JP, et al. Processed allografts and type 1 collagen conduits for repair of peripheral nerve gaps. Muscle Nerve 2009;39:787–99.

Further readings

Abby PA, LaBanc JP, Lupkiewicz S, et al. Fascicular characterization of the human lingual nerve: implications for injury and repair. J Oral Maxillofac Surg 1987;45:43.

Barrows TH. Degradable implant materials: a review of synthetic absorbable polymers and their applications. Clin Mater 1986;1:233.

Brammer JP, Epker BN. Anatomic-histologic survey of the sural nerve: implications for inferior alveolar nerve grafting. J Oral Maxillofac Surg 1988;46:111–7.

Eppley BL, Snyders RV Jr. Microanatomic analysis of the trigeminal nerve and potential nerve graft donor sites. J Oral Maxillofac Surg 1991;49:612–8.

Ginde RM, Gupta RK. In vitro chemical degradation of polyglycolic acid pellets and fibers. J Appl Polym Sci 1987;33:2411.

Herrmann JB, Kelly RJ, Higgins GA. Polyglycolic acid sutures. Laboratory and clinical evaluation of a new absorbable suture material. Arch Surg 1970;100:486–90.

Marmon LM, Vinocur CD, Standiford SB, et al. Evaluation of absorbable polyglycolic acid mesh as a wound support. J Pediatr Surg 1985;20:737–42.

Pogrel MA, McDonald AR, Kaban LB. Gore-Tex tubing as a conduit for repair of lingual and inferior alveolar nerve continuity defects: a preliminary report. J Oral Maxillofac Surg 1998;56:319–21.

Pitta MC, Wolford LM, Mehra P, et al. Use of Gore-Tex tubing as a conduit for inferior alveolar and lingual nerve repair: experience with 6 cases. J Oral Maxillofac Surg 2001;59:493–6.

Siemionow M, Sonmez E. Nerve allograft transplantation: a review. J Reconstr Microsurg 2007;8:511–20.

Trulsson M, Essick GK. Low-threshold mechanoreceptive afferents in the human lingual nerve. J Neurophysiol 1997;77: 737–48.

Terzis JK. Microreconstruction of nerve injuries. Philadelphia: WB Saunders; 1987. p. 227–8.

Wolford LM. Autogenous nerve graft repair of the trigeminal nerve. Oral Maxillofac Surg Clin North Am 1992;4:447–57.

Wessberg GA, Wolford LM, Epker BN. Experiences with microsurgical reconstruction of the inferior alveolar nerve. J Oral Maxillofac Surg 1982;40:651–5.

Sensory Retraining: A Cognitive Behavioral Therapy for Altered Sensation

Ceib Phillips, MPH, PhD[a],*, George Blakey III, DMD[b], Greg K. Essick, DDS, PhD[c]

[a]Department of Orthodontics, CB #7450, University of North Carolina, Chapel Hill, NC 27599, USA
[b]Department of Oral and Maxillofacial Surgery, CB#7450, University of North Carolina, Chapel Hill, NC 27599, USA
[c]Department of Prosthodontics, CB#7450, University of North Carolina, Chapel Hill, NC 27599, USA

Peripheral facial neuropathy

Every year in the United States, millions of people suffer from peripheral neuropathy caused by accidental, compressive, or iatrogenic (eg, surgically associated) injury to the peripheral nervous system. Virtually all of the peripheral nerve injuries to the face occur as a result of nerve compression, stretching, or inflammation of the trigeminal nerve. Elucidation of the mechanisms that influence the rate of peripheral nerve repair after injury is of particular importance for the development of treatments for patients who, after an iatrogenic or other traumatic injury to a peripheral nerve, experience suboptimal recovery of sensory function or the development of neuropathic pain [1,2]. Sensory peripheral nerve injury can result in symptoms that range from a complete or partial loss of sensation (anesthesia or hypoesthesia) to nonpainful tingling sensations (paresthesia), increased sensitivity to touch or pressure with or without numbness or pain (hyperesthesia or dysesthesia), and numbness [3–5]. The extent of sensory impairment, as indicated by stimulus testing measures, has been shown to be reflected in the word descriptors that patients choose to describe their symptoms of altered sensation [6].

Most trigeminal nerve injuries are associated with fracture of the mandible or maxilla. For example, the incidence of somatosensory deficits after facial injuries has been reported as 54.5% in nondisplaced fractures, 88.2% in dislocated fractures, and 100% in fractures with a direct nerve injury [7]. Indeed, after bilateral sagittal split osteotomy, the incidence of nerve injury [8–10] approaches 100%. Using nerve conduction recording methods, the gold standard for assessing the structural integrity of a nerve, one study of 38 trigeminal nerves recorded intraoperatively found that 21 nerves experienced demyelinating injury and 15 axonal damages during the surgery [8]. These injuries result in somatosensory deficit and associated symptoms that most often vary over time and can be unpleasant or painful [4]. Moreover, persistent altered orofacial sensations after a peripheral trigeminal nerve injury often negatively affect patients' lives [11–13]. Those patients who report dysesthetic altered sensations or pain experience the most interference or associated burden in their lives [11,14].

Soft tissue injury and inflammation generally resolve in the first postoperative month after surgery, but the sensory sequelae of the nerve injury may persist for at least 2 years after surgery, which is the longest duration that most studies have observed in patients after treatment [11–17]. Greater than 60% of patients who have undergone bilateral sagittal split osteotomy report persistent altered sensation 6 months after surgery and approximately 20% use descriptors suggestive of unpleasant sensations (dysesthesia), including pain [4,6,11].

This project was supported in part by National Institute of Health grants R01-DE013967 and R01-DE005215.
The authors have nothing to disclose.
* Corresponding author.
E-mail address: Ceib_phillips@dentistry.unc.edu

Afferent nerve recovery and cortical remodeling after nerve injury

After any degree of peripheral nerve injury, a complex of cellular and molecular signaling alterations is immediately initiated, and the quality of functional recovery tightly correlates to the molecular responses that attempt to repair and restore the nerve to its preinjury state. After resolution of inflammation and edema, the sensory deficits can be attributed to anatomic or functional changes within the peripheral nerve or to changes induced in the central nervous system by the nerve injury [18,19]. In general, 3 often temporally overlapping phases may be used to describe this biologic response: the fate determination of the cell body, the active restoration of any loss in the continuity of the proximal and distal segments of the axon and/or reconstitution of axonal diameter and myelination, and the remodeling of the cortical representation of tissues innervated by the damaged axon [20].

Virtually all of the recovery pathway data are derived from transection or crush injuries in animal models, in which case axonal regrowth, reconstitution, and remyelination are essential, but it is reasonable to assume that nontransecting injuries activate similar pathways [21]. Axonal damage is often severe even without transection, requiring reconnection of axonal sprouts to target tissues, reconstitution of axonal damage, and remyelination of myelinated afferents [8]. Once the fate of the injured neuron is set, the surviving cell body actively intensifies its transcriptional machinery for the heightened synthesis of structural proteins for axonal repair and regeneration, if required, and restoration of electrical conduction from the tissues [22–26].

Finally, injury-associated alterations in the peripheral nerve induce changes in neural substrates at subcortical and cortical levels within the central nervous system [27,28]. The underlying mechanisms of this central plasticity are largely unknown, but a heightened excitability is often observed in cortical regions that remodel in response to nerve injury [20]. In a sense, neuroplasticity reflects the competition between afferent inputs for connections in the sensory cortex. Microelectrodes implanted in the cortex and subcortical relay stations on the sensory path between the face and the cortex in rats showed new responses to other facial areas within minutes of the deactivation of their usual sensory input [29].

This cortical reorganization is reflected in the altered symptoms that are experienced by individuals after sensory nerve injuries. In the normal state, stimulation of the face or lips by contact with the external environment stimulates the sensory receptors, and a profile of neural impulses is elicited. These impulses affect the sensory cortex and are associated with previous memory of experiences. After a nerve injury, the same contact (the same stimulus) with the external world elicits a different, altered profile of neural impulses [30].

Sensory retraining background

Sensory retraining (also referred to as sensory reeducation) is a cognitive behavioral therapy technique that helps the patient with a nerve injury to meaningfully interpret the altered profile or neural impulses reaching his/her conscious level after the altered sensation area has been stimulated [30]. Moreover, the repetitive neural input from sensory retraining exercises can produce plastic changes in the somatosensory cortex via the same mechanisms underlying those evoked by altered input from the nerve damage. This reorganization through retraining can compensate, in part, for some of the impairments associated with nerve injury [31–37].

Animal studies have shown that behavioral sensory training alters the central neural representation of the involved skin sites, alters the response of individual somatosensory cortical cells to tactile stimulation, increases synapse to neuron ratios, and improves behavioral function after induced brain damage more than simple repetitive exercise [38–44]. Neuroimaging studies indicate that similar changes occur in human subjects after sensory denervation and sensory training [45]. Sensory re-education or retraining results in somatosensory cortical maps that exhibit higher sensory resolution and greater topographic organization, which facilitate better interpretation of sensory inputs. In contrast to the central neural changes, sensory retraining does not alter the course of nerve regeneration or the absolute thresholds to touch [39,46–48] but does improve both the patient's cognitive and adaptive responses to stimulation of the affected skin region [12,30,49–51].

Although improvement has been reported when retraining is not initiated soon after the injury, reorganization of the cortex after changes in peripheral input happens quite quickly. Persistent chronic altered sensation may result in irreversible cortical changes. One of the goals of retraining is to avoid, minimize, or modulate the central functional reorganization [52].

The process of sensory retraining can be likened to the brain learning a new language in progressive phases of difficulty. Initially, use of the words is slow, challenging, and error prone. With time and practice, verbal fluency may be acquired. Unfortunately, no research has been conducted to determine the optimal number of phases or the exercises required to obtain the maximum benefit to patients with orofacial nerve injuries.

Historically, in the early phase of sensory retraining (Box 1), the intent is to reeducate constant versus moving touch perceptions. That is, a patient must relearn what constant touch feels like compared with moving touch and where on the skin the touch is actually occurring. In the early phase, a greater stimulus intensity may be necessary for the patient to differentiate constant from moving touch, but the intensity should never be so great as to evoke pain. If hyperesthesia or dysesthesia occurs, desensitization with gentle stroking using different textures or gentle tapping is recommended [53–56]. In the late phase of retraining (see Box 1), the intent is to reeducate the directionality of movement perceptions of the patient. For example, is the movement of an external object across the skin from left to right or right to left?

For orofacial sensory retraining, an important component of the retraining exercises is the visual feedback provided by performing the exercises in front of a mirror. This visual feedback elicits 2 different sensory events, the sensation of the brush on the facial skin and the sight of the brush on the face. Recent experimental studies have shown that viewing a body surface can directly enhance tactile perception and detection [57,58] even when the touch is not physical but a mirrored reflection [59,60]. The frequency with which the exercises are performed each day is much more important than the length of time spent at any given time. It may be that encouraging patients to perform orofacial sensory retraining exercises with a small handheld mirror for a short period of time, perhaps 1 to 2 minutes, 4 to 6 times per day, would be as or more effective than a longer less frequent protocol.

Both the potential for acquiring the "second language" of sensory retraining and its effectiveness decreases with age [49,50,61], varies with the verbal learning capacity and visuospatial cognitive skills of the patient, and depends on motivation and positive reinforcement [45].

Sensory retraining as a rehabilitative approach has been used extensively over the past several decades for patients who had nerve injuries affecting the hand. The emphasis of the sensory retraining exercises for patients with hand injury and those with stroke has been to teach the patients to interpret the percepts of objects manipulated by the fingers in a meaningful and functional way [30,53,62–64]. Patients with hand injury learn to recognize and discriminate the shapes of small objects (various buttons, coins, and keys). Patients gain the ability to button their own shirt and identify shapes without visual cues (eg, a key vs a coin). Although the touch percepts produced by the objects remain

---

Box 1. General concepts of sensory retraining

Two Phases
 Early phase: constant versus moving touch
 Late phase: directionality
Frequency: 3 or 4 times a day for a couple of minutes
General Strategies:
 Quiet surroundings. Concentration is important.
 Use stimulus (cloth, cosmetic brush, cotton swab), not finger. Using a finger would create 2 sets of sensory information for the patient which would confuse the already distorted sensory picture.
Components of Retraining
 1) Observation of touch/movement. For the face, it is critical to use visual feedback via a mirror.
 2) Concentration on perception of touch/movement, with eyes closed to combine the mental with the visual picture.
 3) Repeat observation for visual confirmation of touch/movement.
 4) Verbalize the touch/movement being performed and what it feels like.
 5) Incorporate unaffected areas using the same procedure so that the sensation on the 2 sides may be compared.

abnormal after retraining, patients become more comfortable with, and accepting of, the situation because the percepts are no longer functionally disabling.

The same therapeutic approach, incorporating meaningful and graded stimuli, active participation, and accurate feedback, has successfully been used to improve tactile and proprioceptive discrimination after a stroke [65,66] and recovery of function in people with brain damage [67]. An adaptation of sensory reeducation, mirror box therapy, has successfully been used with patients with phantom limb pain [68], hemiparesis after stroke [69], and complex regional pain syndrome type 1 [70]. Patients have regained functionality and mobility with reduced pain and evidence of cortical reorganization of the primary somatosensory cortex that paralleled their clinical improvement [71].

Sensory retraining for altered orofacial sensation

The question of whether sensory retraining exercises could be used effectively with patients with altered orofacial sensation was first raised in the literature by Gregg [72] in 1992. In 2001, Meyer and Rath [53] presented a retrospective review of 372 patients who had had a microsurgical repair for a nerve injury after 1981 and for whom at least an 18-month postsurgical follow-up was available. A nonrandom sample of patients had been given facial sensory exercise instructions that incorporated some of the early stage components of sensory retraining, with the expectation that sensory retraining would help patients with altered oral-facial sensation after nerve injury by (1) improving patients' ability to interpret lip/chin sensations and movements, (2) improving perioral motor function subjectively and objectively, and (3) lessening the objectionable impression of numb/paresthetic sensations in the lip and chin by decreasing the subjective differences between affected and unaffected skin areas. The percentage of patients who achieved a useful sensory recovery on the Medical Research Council Scale, a clinical assessment, did not differ between those who did and did not receive instructions regarding facial sensory exercises. However, those patients who received instructions reached their final level of sensory recovery much sooner, on average 3 months earlier [53].

To assess the efficacy of sensory retraining for facial altered sensation, a multicenter, double-blind, parallel, 2-arm stratified block randomized clinical trial (RCT) was conducted at an academic center and a community-based center with enrollment of 191 subjects. The intent was to assess whether the magnitude and duration of patient-reported burden from altered sensation was lessened when facial sensory retraining exercises were performed in conjunction with standard opening exercises than when the opening exercises were performed alone. The subjects were patients with a developmental disharmony who were scheduled for a bilateral sagittal split osteotomy with or without a maxillary osteotomy. Just as third molar extraction is an excellent model for analgesic pain studies, candidates for orthognathic surgery constitute an ideal subject group for the investigation of novel putative therapies for nerve injury-associated altered sensation. Baseline data can be obtained before altered sensation develops (presurgically), and these baseline responses can be compared subsequently with those obtained immediately after nervy injury and during the recovery process. Because the surgery is elective, patients are typically healthy, young adults without preexisting conditions or complications that can make interpretation of therapeutic effect more difficult.

The emphasis on patient report in the RCT was motivated by 2 factors: (1) the assumption that sensory retraining would not affect nerve recovery and therefore basic sensory testing measures of nerve function and (2) the recognition of the different functions of the sensory innervations to the facial versus digital skin. The terminal distribution of the inferior alveolar nerve, the mental nerve, innervates skin functionally more like the back of the hand (radial nerve) than the palm side of the hand (median and ulnar nerves) [73]. Thus, the skin of the hairy lower lip and chin of the face deform in response to movements during function, and as such, the evoked neural discharge serves a proprioceptive role including a conscious awareness of facial expressions [74,75].

The sensory retraining protocol in the RCT had 3, time-dependent levels of instructions that were given to patients at 1 week, 1 month (4 to 6 weeks), and 3 months after surgery. The time points were selected based on the use of these instructions in clinical studies of the impact of sensory reeducation in patients with an injured median or ulnar nerve [64] and in clinical studies of sensory impairment in patients after orthognathic surgery [76–79]. The 3 levels of sensory retraining were designed to increasingly challenge patients congruent with the early and late phases of sensory education used for the hand: constant versus moving touch, orientation of moving touch, and direction of moving

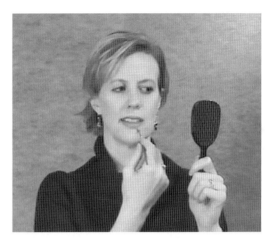

Fig. 1. Screen shot of sensory retraining exercise instruction: simple touch and stroke with cosmetic brush (motion training) and mirror. Three videos demonstrating each exercise at each level are available online within this article at www.oralmaxsurgeryatlas.theclinics.com, March 2011 issue. (The screen shot and videos are © Video Services of the Center for Instructional Technology at the University of North Carolina, Chapel Hill, NC.)

touch (Fig. 1, Table 1). (Three videos (Videos 1–3) demonstrating each exercise at each level are available online within this article at www.oralmaxsurgeryatlas.theclinics.com, March 2011 issue. The videos were produced by Video Services of the Center for Instructional Technology at the University of North Carolina. Written instructions provided to subjects and copies of the instructional tapes are available from the corresponding author upon request.)

Consistent with the anecdotal reports, the patients in this clinical trial who received the sensory retraining exercise instruction were less likely to report a problem related to unusual feelings on the face, loss of lip sensitivity, or numbness at 3 and 6 months after surgery than subjects who received standard opening exercises only [12,80]. At 6 months, subjects in the opening-only exercise group were almost twice as likely as those in the sensory retraining group to report a problem with altered sensation [12,80]. In addition to patient-reported outcomes, 2-point perception, 2-point discrimination, and contact detection thresholds were measured as secondary outcomes. The sensory retraining patients were more adept at perceiving touch (Fig. 2), indicating accommodation, even though there was no improvement in the ability to discriminate 2 distinct points of contact from 1 (nerve recovery) [46].

The positive effect of the sensory retraining persisted even after the exercise protocol was completed. Although the likelihood that a subject would report altered sensation steadily decreased in both groups over a 2-year follow-up, the difference between the groups was relatively consistent. Even at 2 years after surgery, patients who received only the opening exercises were about 2 times more likely to report an altered sensation than patients who used the sensory retraining exercises after surgery (Fig. 3) [49],

Table 1
Synopsis of instructions given to the opening-only exercise group and the sensory retraining group at each of the 3 training sessions. Subjects in the sensory retraining group also were instructed and asked to perform the opening exercises

Visit	Opening exercises (3x/day)	Sensory retraining exercises (2x/day)
1 week	Simple open/close and side/side using jaw muscles only	Alternate simple touch and stroke with cosmetic brush (motion training)
	Movement until discomfort only not till pain	Feedback from mirror
	Hold and relax	Visualization with eyes closed
1 month	Hold and relax	Alternate up/down and side/side strokes (orientation training)
	Finger stretch for simple open/close	
	Movement until discomfort only not till pain	Feedback from mirror
		Visualization with eyes closed
3 months	If opening ≥35 mm	Alternate up→down and down→up strokes (directionality training)
	Occasionally repeat exercises	
	If opening <35 mm	Feedback from mirror
	Increase frequency of exercises	Visualization with eyes closed

From Phillips C, Essick G, Preisser JS, et al. Sensory retraining following orthognathic surgery: effect on patient perception of altered sensation. J Oral Maxillofac Surg 2007;65:1162–73; with permission.

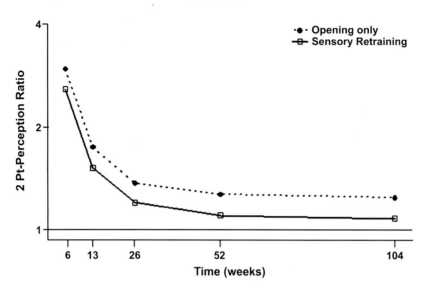

Fig. 2. Estimates of the adjusted mean impairment ratio in 2-point perception for subjects who did and did not receive sensory retraining exercises. The lower 2-point perception impairment ratio, on average, for the sensory retraining group indicates that this group was able to report 2 distinct points at shorter separations than the opening-only group. The y-axis is scaled logarithmically. A value of 1 indicates a return to presurgical value.

and patients in the sensory retraining group were less likely to report interference in daily life activities from numbness or loss of lip sensitivity (Fig. 4) [50]. This difference between the 2 exercise groups seems to be related to the difference in how the "retrained" individual experienced or interpreted tactile stimuli rather than any difference in nerve recovery or repair [46,47].

The primary efficacy results at 6 months and the longer-term recovery analyses at 24 months indicate that for patients who experience an acute nerve injury, as is highly likely during a mandibular osteotomy, the simple, noninvasive sensory retraining facial exercises, which require only an inexpensive cosmetic brush and a mirror, are an effective cognitive behavioral therapy to promote accommodation to a sensory deficit on the face. Perhaps, the desired outcome for retrained patients was best stated by Callahan [54]: "If sensory re-education results in a person's increased ability to better enjoy the tactile sensations of everyday living, then reeducation has been meaningful and successful."

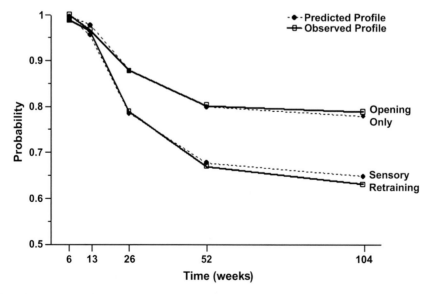

Fig. 3. Estimated and observed likelihood of the presence of altered sensations for subjects who did and did not receive sensory retraining exercises after controlling for psychological distress and age. (*From* Phillips C, Kim S, Essick G, et al. Sensory retraining following orthognathic surgery: Effect on patient report of the presence of altered sensation. Am J Ortho Dentofac Orthop 2009;136:788–94; with permission.)

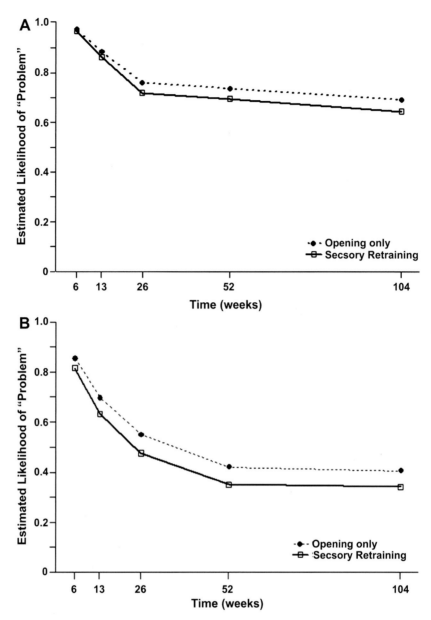

Fig. 4. Estimated likelihood of a subject reporting at least some problem or interference in daily life after controlling for psychological distress and age for subjects who did and did not receive sensory retraining exercises. (*A*) Problem associated with numbness. (*B*) Problem associated with loss of lip sensitivity.

Summary

1) Sensory retraining teaches the patient to ignore or blot out postinjury unpleasant orofacial sensations to optimally tune into and decipher the weakened and damaged signals from the tissues.
2) Sensory retraining is a simple, inexpensive, noninvasive exercise program, which initiated shortly after injury, can lessen the objectionable impression of orofacial altered sensations.
3) Sensory retraining exercises are most effective in decreasing the perceived burden associated with hypoesthetic orofacial altered sensations.

Acknowledgments

We wish to thank Dr Myron Tucker and the staff at Oral and Maxillofacial Surgery in Charlotte, NC, for their participation in the RCT.

Supplementary data

Supplementary data related to this article can be found online at doi:10.1016/j.cxom.2010.11.006.

References

[1] Kawasaki Y, Xu ZZ, Wang X, et al. Distinct roles of matrix metalloproteases in the early- and late-phase development of neuropathic pain. Nat Med 2008;14:331–6.
[2] Treede RD, Jensen TS, Campbell JN, et al. Neuropathic pain. Redefinition and a grading system for clinical and research purposes. Neurology 2008;70:1630–5.
[3] Available at: http://www.neuropathy.org/site/PageServer?pagename=About_Facts. Accessed September 29, 2008.
[4] Phillips C, Essick G, Zuniga J, et al. Qualitative descriptors used by patients following orthognathic surgery to portray altered sensation. J Oral Maxillofac Surg 2006;64:1751–60.
[5] Meyer-Rosberg K, Kvarnstrom A, Kinnman E, et al. Peripheral neuropathic pain-a multidimensional burden for patients. Eur J Pain 2001;5:3779–89.
[6] Essick GK, Phillips C, Turvey TA, et al. Facial altered sensation and sensory impairment after orthognathic surgery. Int J Oral Maxillofac Surg 2007;36:577–82.
[7] Renzi G, Carboni A, Perugini M, et al. Posttraumatic trigeminal nerve impairment: a prospective analysis of recovery patterns in a series of 103 consecutive facial fractures. J Oral Maxillofac Surg 2004;62:1341–6.
[8] Jääskeläinen SK, Teerijoki-Oksa T, Virtanen A, et al. Sensory regeneration following intraoperatively verified trigeminal nerve injury. Neurology 2004;62:1951–7.
[9] Nakagawa K, Ueki K, Takatsuka S, et al. Somatosensory-evoked potential to evaluate the trigeminal nerve after sagittal split osteotomy. Oral Surg Oral Med Oral Pathol Oral Radiol Endod 2001;91:146–52.
[10] Jones DL, Wolford LM. Intraoperative recording of trigeminal evoked potentials during orthognathic surgery. Int J Adult Orthodon Orthognath Surg 1990;5:167–74.
[11] Phillips C, Essick G, Blakey G 3rd, et al. Relationship between patients' perceptions of postsurgical sequelae and altered sensations after bilateral sagittal split osteotomy. J Oral Maxillofac Surg 2007;65:597–607.
[12] Phillips C, Essick G, Preisser JS, et al. Sensory retraining after orthognathic surgery: effect on patients' perception of altered sensation. J Oral Maxillofac Surg 2007;65:1162–73.
[13] Phillips C, Proffitt WR. Psychosocial aspects of dentofacial deformity and its treatment. In: Proffit WR, White RP, Sarver DM, editors. Contemporary treatment of dentofacial deformity. New York: Mosby; 2003. p. 69–90.
[14] Harvey WS, Phillips CL, Essick GK. Neurosensory impairment and patient perception of recovery following orthognathic surgery. J Dent Res 2001;80(special issue):187.
[15] Kehlet H, Jensen TS, Woolf CJ. Persistent postsurgical pain: risk factors and prevention. Lancet 2006;367:1618–825.
[16] Westermark A, Bystedt H, von Konow L. Inferior alveolar nerve function after mandibular osteotomies. Br J Oral Maxillofac Surg 1998;36:425–8.
[17] Westermark A, Englesson L, Bongenhielm U. Neurosensory function after sagittal split osteotomy of the mandible: a comparison between subjective evaluation and objective assessment. Int J Adult Orthodon Orthognath Surg 1999;14:268–75.
[18] Essick G. Psychophysical assessment of patients with posttraumatic neuropathic trigeminal pain. J Orofac Pain 2004;18:345–54.
[19] Becerra L, Morris S, Bazes S, et al. Trigeminal neuropathic pain alters responses in CNS circuits to mechanical (brush) and thermal (cold and heat) stimuli. J Neurosci 2006;26:10646–57.
[20] Navarro X, Vivó M, Valero-Cabré A. Neural plasticity after peripheral nerve injury and regeneration. Prog Neurobiol 2007;82:163–201.
[21] Atusmi Y, Imai T, Matsumoto K, et al. Effects of different types of injury to the inferior alveolar nerve on the behavior of Schwann cells during the regeneration of periodontal nerve fibers of rat incisor. Arch Histol Cytol 2000;63:43–54.
[22] Abe N, Cavalli V. Nerve injury signaling. Curr Opin Neurobiol 2008;18:276–83.
[23] Hanz S, Fainzilber M. Retrograde signaling in injured nerve-the axon reaction revisited. J Neurochem 2006;99:13–9.
[24] Mandolesi G, Madeddu F, Bozzi Y, et al. Acute physiological response of mammalian central neurons to axotomy: ionic regulation and electrical activity. Faseb J 2004;18:1934–6.
[25] Boyd JG, Gordon T. Neurotrophic factors and their receptors in axonal regeneration and functional recovery after peripheral nerve injury. Mol Neurobiol 2003;27:277–324.
[26] Herdegen T, Skene P, Bahr M. The c-Jun transcription factor–bipotential mediator of neuronal death, survival and regeneration. Trends Neurosci 1997;20:227–31.
[27] Kaas JH, Collins CE. Anatomic and functional reorganization of somatosensory cortex in mature primates after peripheral nerve and spinal cord injury. Adv Neurol 2003;93:87–95.
[28] Wall JT, Xu J, Wang X. Human brain plasticity: an emerging view of the multiple substrates and mechanisms that cause cortical changes and related sensory dysfunctions after injuries of sensory inputs from the body. Brain Res Rev 2002;39:181–215.
[29] Faggin BM, Nguyen KT, Nicolelis MA. Immediate and simultanous sensory reorganization at cortical and subcortical levels of the somatosensory system. Proc Natl Acad Sci U S A 1997;94:9428–533.
[30] Dellon AL. Re-education of sensation. In: Dellon AL, editor. Evaluation of sensibility and re-education of sensation in the hand. Baltimore (MD): John D Lucas; 1988. p. 203–46.
[31] Dubner R, Ruda MA. Activity-dependent neuronal plasticity following tissue injury and inflammation [Review]. Trends Neurosci 1992;15(3):96–103.

[32] Essick GK. Comprehensive clinical evaluation of perioral sensory function. Oral Maxillofac Surg Clin North Am 1992; 4(2):503–26.
[33] Woolf CJ, Walters ET. Common patterns of plasticity contributing to nociceptive sensitization in mammals and Aplysia [Review] [60 refs]. Trends Neurosci 1991;14(2):74–8.
[34] Gregg JM. Studies of traumatic neuralgias in the maxillofacial region: surgical pathology and neural mechanisms. J Oral Maxillofac Surg 1990;48(3):228–37 [discussion: 238–9].
[35] Cusick CG, Wall JT, Whiting JH, et al. Temporal progression of cortical reorganization following nerve injury. Brain Res 1990;537(1–2):355–8.
[36] Merzenich MM, Recanzone G, Jenkins WM, et al. Cortical representational plasticity. In: Rakic P, Singer W, editors. Neurobiology of Neocortex. Chichester (NY): John Wiley & Sons; 1988. p. 41–67.
[37] Wall JT, Kaas JH, Sur M, et al. Functional reorganization in somatosensory cortical areas 3b and 1 of adult monkeys after median nerve repair: possible relationships to sensory recovery in humans. J Neurosci 1986;6:218–23.
[38] Florence SL, Boydston LA, Hackett TA, et al. Sensory enrichment after peripheral nerve injury restores cortical, not thalamic, receptive field organization. Eur J Neurosci 2001;13:1755–66.
[39] Jones TA, Ghu CJ, Grande LA, et al. Motor skills training enhances lesion-induced structural plasticity in the motor cortex of adult rats. J Neurosci 1999;19(22):10153–63.
[40] Jones TA, Hawrylak N, Klintsova AY, et al. Brain damage, behavior, rehabilitation, recovery, and brain plasticity. Ment Retard Dev Disabil Res Rev 1998;4:231–7.
[41] Recanzone GH, Jenkins WM, Hradek GT, et al. Progressive improvement in discriminative abilities in adult owl monkeys performing a tactile frequency discrimination task. J Neurophysiol 1992;67:1015–30.
[42] Recanzone GH, Merzenich MM, Jenkins WM, et al. Topographic reorganization of the hand representation in cortical area 3b of owl monkeys trained in a frequency-discrimination task. J Neurophysiol 1992;67:1031–55.
[43] Recanzone GH, Merzenich MM, Schreiner CE. Changes in the distributed temporal response properties of SI cortical neurons reflect improvements in performance on a temporally based tactile discrimination task. J Neurophysiol 1992; 67:1071–92.
[44] Jenkins WM, Merzenich MM, Ochs MT, et al. Functional reorganization of primary somatosensory cortex in adult owl monkeys after behaviorally controlled tactile stimulation. J Neurophysiol 1990;63:82–104.
[45] Lundborg G. Nerve injury and repair: a challenge to the plastic brain. J Peripher Nerv Syst 2003;8:209.
[46] Essick GK, Phillips C, Zuniga J. Effect of facial sensory retraining on sensory thresholds. J Dent Res 2007;86:571–5.
[47] Essick GK, Phillips C, Kim SK, et al. Sensory retraining following orthognathic surgery: effect on threshold measures of sensory function. J Oral Rehabil 2009;36(6):415–26.
[48] Bell-Krotoski J, Weinstein S, Weinstein C. Testing sensibility, including touch-pressure, two-point discrimination, point localization, and vibration. J Hand Ther 1993;6:114–23.
[49] Phillips C, Kim S, Essick G, et al. Sensory retraining following orthognathic surgery: effect on patient report of the presence of altered sensation. Am J Orthod Dentofacial Orthop 2009;136(6):788–94.
[50] Phillips C, Kim S, Tucker M, et al. Sensory retraining: burden in daily life related to altered sensation after orthognathic surgery, a randomized clinical trial. Orthod Craniofac Res 2010;13(3):169–78.
[51] Daniele HR, Aguado L. Early compensatory sensory re-education. J Reconstr Microsurg 2003;19:107–10.
[52] Rosen B, Lundborg G. Sensory re-education after nerve repair: Aspects of timing. Handchir Mikrochir Plast Chir 2004;36: 8–12.
[53] Meyer RA, Rath EM. Sensory rehabilitation after trigeminal nerve injury or nerve repair. Atlas Oral Maxillofac Surg Clin North Am 2001;13:365.
[54] Callahan AD. Methods of compensation and re-education for sensory dysfunction. In: Hunter JM, Mackin EJ, Callahan AD, editors. Rehabilitation of the Hand. St Louis (MO): Mosby; 1995. p. 611–21.
[55] Imai H, Tajima T, Natsumi Y. Successful reeducation of functional sensibility after median nerve repair at the wrist. J Hand Surg 1991;16:60.
[56] Waylett-Rendall J. Sensibility evaluation and rehabilitation. Orthop Clin North Am 1988;19:43.
[57] Fiorio M, Haggard P. Viewing the body prepares the brain for touch: effects of TMS over somatosensory cortex. Eur J Neurosci 2005;22:773–7.
[58] Taylor-Clarke M, Kennett S, Haggard P. Vision modulates somatosensory cortical processing. Curr Biol 2002;12:233–6.
[59] Ro T, Wallace R, Hagedorn J, et al. Visual enhancing of tactile perception in the posterior parietal cortex. J Cogn Neurosci 2004;16:24–30.
[60] Sathian K, Greenspan AI, Wolf SL. Doing it with mirrors: a case study of a novel approach to neurorehabilitation-Neurorehabil Neural Repair 2000;14:73–6.
[61] Lundborg G, Rosen B. Sensory relearning after nerve repair. Lancet 2001;358:809–10.
[62] Shieh SJ, Chiu HO, Lee JW, et al. Evaluation of the effectiveness of sensory reeducation following digital replantation and revascularization. Microsurgery 1995;16:578–82.
[63] Wei FC, Ma HS. Delayed sensory reeducation after toe-to-hand transfer. Microsurgery 1995;16:583–5.
[64] Wynn Parry CB, Slater M. Sensory re-education after median nerve lesions. Hand 1976;8:250–7.
[65] Carey LM, Matyas TA, Oke LE. Sensory loss in stroke patients: effective training of tactile and proprioceptive discrimination. Arch Phys Med Rehabil 1993;74:602–11.
[66] Yekutiel M. Sensory loss after stroke. In: Yekutiel M, editor. Sensory re-education of the hand after stroke. Philadelphia (PA): Whurr Pub; 2005. p. 14–28.
[67] Bach-y-Rita B. Brain plasticity as a basis for therapeutic procedures. In: Bach-y-Rita P, editor. Recovery of function: theoretical considerations for brain injury rehabilitation. Vienna (Austria): Hans Huber; 1980. p. 225–63.
[68] Ramachandran VS. Phantom limbs and neural plasticity. Arch Neurol 2000;57:317–20.
[69] Altschuler E, Wisdom SB, Stone L, et al. Rehabilitation of hemiparesis alfter stroke with a mirror. Lancet 1999;353:235.

[70] McCabe CS, Haigh RC, Ring EF, et al. A controlled pilot study of the utility of mirror visual feedback in the treatment of complex regional pain syndrome (type 1). Rheumatology (Oxford) 2003;42:97–101.
[71] Mailhofner C, Handwerker HO, Neundorfe B, et al. Cortical reorganization during recovery from complex regional pain syndrome. Neurology 2004;63:693–701.
[72] Gregg JM. Nonsurgical management of traumatic trigeminal neuralgias and sensory neuropathies. Oral Maxillofac Surg Clin North Am 1992;4:375–92.
[73] Trulsson M, Essick GK. Low-threshold mechanoreceptive afferents in the human lingual nerve. J Neurophysiol 1997;77:737.
[74] Edin BB, Johansson N. Skin strain patterns provide kinaesthetic information to the human central nervous system. J Physiol (Lond) 1995;1:243.
[75] Gandevia SC, Phegan CML. Perceptual distortions of the human body image produced by local anaesthesia, pain and cutaneous stimulation. J Physiol (Lond) 1999;2:609.
[76] Yoshida T, Nagamine T, Kobayashi T, et al. Impairment of the inferior alveolar nerve after sagittal split osteotomy. J Craniomaxillofac Surg 1989;17:271.
[77] Karas ND, Boyd SB, Sinn DP. Recovery of neurosensory function following orthognathic surgery. J Oral Maxillofac Surg 1990;48:124.
[78] Van Boven RW, Johnson KO. A psychophysical study of the mechanisms of sensory recovery following nerve injury in humans. Brain 1994;117:149.
[79] Fridrich KL, Holton TJ, Pansegrau KJ, et al. Neurosensory recovery following the mandibular bilateral sagittal split osteotomy. J Oral Maxillofac Surg 1995;53:1300.
[80] Preisser JS, Phillips C, Perin J, et al. Regression models for patient-reported measures having ordered categories recorded on multiple occasions. Community Dent Oral Epidemiol 2010. [Epub ahead of print].

Advances in Bioengineered Conduits for Peripheral Nerve Regeneration

Martin B. Steed, DDS[a],*, Vivek Mukhatyar, BS[b], Chandra Valmikinathan, PhD[c], Ravi V. Bellamkonda, PhD[d]

[a]Division of Oral and Maxillofacial Surgery, Department of Surgery, Emory University School of Medicine, 1365 Clifton Road, Suite 2300 B, Atlanta, GA 30322, USA
[b]Wallace H. Coulter Department of Biomedical Engineering, Georgia Institute of Technology/Emory University, 3108 UA Whitaker Building, 313 Ferst Drive Northeast, Atlanta, GA 30332-0535, USA
[c]Wallace H. Coulter Department of Biomedical Engineering, Georgia Institute of Technology/Emory University, 2245 UA Whitaker Building, 313 Ferst Drive Northeast, Atlanta, GA 30332-0535, USA
[d]Neurological Biomaterials & Therapeutics, Wallace H. Coulter Department of Biomedical Engineering, Georgia Institute of Technology/Emory University, 3108 UA Whitaker Building, 313 Ferst Drive Northeast, Atlanta, GA 30332-0535, USA

Peripheral nerve injury and regeneration in the maxillofacial region remain significant clinical problems. Peripheral nerves, including the inferior alveolar and lingual nerves, possess a limited ability to regenerate after traumatic injury. The quality of this regeneration depends on several factors. These include the size and type of injury, location, and the age of the patient. Healing after nerve trauma is complicated, partly because mature neurons do not replicate. Under the right conditions, however, axons can regenerate across relatively long nerve gaps generated due to injury or resection of tumors, reconnecting with distal stump and eventually reestablishing functional contacts. Those nerves that do not spontaneously restore their function require microsurgical end-to-end coaptation of proximal and distal nerve segments to produce a tension free repair. When surgical repair is required for a transected nerve, or a neuroma requiring excision, higher success rates have been seen with direct repair rather than through the use of grafts. Better results are obtained when the nerves are purely motor or purely sensory and when the amount of intraneural connective tissue is relatively small. For optimal nerve regeneration after repair, nerve stumps must be properly prepared, aligned without tension, and repaired atraumatically with minimal tissue damage and minimal number of sutures. When primary repair cannot be performed without undue tension, nerve grafting or tubulization techniques are required.

The current gold standard for bridging nerve gaps is nerve autografting. Autologous nerve grafts fulfill the criteria for an ideal nerve conduit, because they provide a permissive and stimulating scaffold, including Schwann cell basal laminae, neurotrophic factors, and adhesion molecules. The disadvantages of this technique include donor site morbidity, size mismatch between injured nerve and graft nerve diameter, neuroma formation at the donor site, and even in the best-case scenarios, incomplete recovery. Increasing evidence suggests that the modality of the donor nerve may influence regeneration, with mixed nerves or purely motor donor nerves having better outcomes than commonly used sensory nerves such as sural nerves. In addition, peripheral nerves might also express inhibitory proteoglycans such as chondroitin sulfate proteoglycans.

These limitations of autografting have encouraged the search for alternative means of nerve gap reconstruction. These have included nerve allografts and biologic and artificial conduits. Achieving better clinical outcomes in the future depends greatly upon simultaneous advancements in microsurgical technique, but perhaps more importantly, translation of molecular biology and

The authors have nothing to disclose.
* Corresponding author.
E-mail address: msteed@emory.edu

bioengineering discoveries into clinical practice. The field of peripheral nerve research is a dynamically developing arena, and recent concentration has focused on sophisticated approaches tested at the basic science level. To date, much of the research effort has focused on nerve guidance channels (NGCs) to enhance regeneration across nerve gaps. The purpose of this article is to illustrate recent advances in artificial NGCs and discuss the variables that may be manipulated to enhance the efficacy of scaffolds designed for peripheral nerve regeneration, which may have a dramatic clinical impact on peripheral trigeminal nerve injury in the future.

Artificial conduits

Over the past 25 years the concept of an NGC has evolved from a tool to investigate nerve regeneration to a device that is being used clinically in patients as an alternative to autografts. Their use has been mostly limited to the repair of small defects (<3 cm) in small-caliber digital nerves. There have been reports of use in the maxillofacial region, but few outcome studies at present. Initial clinical trigeminal nerve case series showed poor outcomes with the use of Gore-Tex conduits for inferior alveolar and lingual nerve repair. Possible improvement upon this nonresorbable material with the use of a polyglycolic acid conduit filled with heparin has been proposed. Presently there are several tubes being marketed including Neurotube (Synovis), Neurolac (Ascension), SaluBridge (SaluMedica), and NeuraGen (Integra). While these NGCs have been shown to enhance regeneration across nerve gaps when compared with no intervention, guidance channels rarely approach the performance of autografts when the gaps are 10 mm or longer in a rat model. Although approved for human use, the efficacy for each is limited to the repair of short defects (<3 cm) of small-caliber nerves. The basic design of these tubes has been similar, namely a hollow tube in which the two ends of the nerve are inserted at either end. They differ, however, in the composition and properties of the biomaterial from which they are made. Currently, there is little information as to which tube provides better clinical outcomes in the repair of small nerve gaps.

In the last decade, artificial NGCs have been produced using various natural (collagen) and synthetic, nonbiodegradable polymers (silicone) and biodegradable polymers, including poly lactic acid and polycaprolactone (PGA, PCL, hydrogel). Multiple modification techniques have been developed to obtain porous and nonporous NGCs, incorporate electrically active channels into the channels, or utilize bioactive fillers within the lumen of the NGCs. The current trend in peripheral nerve research and tissue engineering is the realization of biomimetic NGCs providing topological, haptotactic, and chemotactic signaling to cells, respectively by surface functionalization with cell binding domains, the use of internal oriented fibers and the sustained release of neurotrophic factors.

Generally, NGCs can be categorized by whether they are degradable or nondegradable, and by the nature of additional cues that are presented within the lumens of NGCs to promote axonal regeneration.

Nonbiodegradable Materials as NGCs

Silicone NGCs have been used historically for peripheral nerve repair. They have been widely employed to study NGC fillers, as they are nonbiodegradable and not permeable to large molecules. Disadvantages of the use of nondegradable NGCs include chronic foreign body reaction, inflexibility, and lack of stability. Particularly, the inflammatory response of silicone NGCs may lead to fibrotic capsule formation around the guide and consequent nerve compression. Alterations in the blood–nerve barrier occur, followed by demyelination of the nerve fibers. Silicone tubes used as NGCs clinically must be removed for a successful outcome.

Biodegradable Synthetic Materials as NGCs

Recent research has been focused on biodegradable NGCs. Biodegradable NGCs should ideally not be toxic or elicit an immunologic response and be able to bear the stresses of the surgical procedure (handling and suturing) and implantation time (due to patient movements). Various different synthetic biomaterials have been used in the fabrication of NGCs, mostly polymers of lactic and glycolic acid and capralactone through various fabrication techniques. Both the material composition and the fabrication technique have great influence on the physical properties of the NGC for entubulation repair; these properties include permeability, swelling, and degradation behavior.

Permeability of a NGC is an important property, as nutrients and oxygen need to diffuse to the site of regeneration before revascularization and may influence the formation of fibrin matrix in the initial stage of regeneration. It should allow for the exchange of fluids between the regenerating environment and avoid the build-up of pressure due to fluid retention. At the same time, the pore dimension has to be small enough to prevent infiltration of scar-forming fibroblasts that could alter the regeneration process. Different fabrication techniques can make NGCs permeable including cutting holes in the wall of the tube, rolling of meshes, adding salt or sugar crystals, which are leached after fabrication, or by injection molding solvent evaporation. The permeability of an NGC can be closely related to the crystallinity of the material. As the crystalline phase is inaccessible to water and other permeable molecules, both biodegradation and permeability decrease with increasing crystallinity degree. Permeability also depends upon the hydrophilic properties of the material, which can be measured from the contact angle of a drop of water on the material. It is not known whether the extended regeneration with the use of permeable chambers is due to:

Metabolic exchange across the tube wall (diffusion of nutrients such as glucose, oxygen, and elimination of waste products)
Diffusion into the guide lumen of growth or trophic factors generated in the external environment (wound healing factors)
Retention of growth or trophic factors secreted by the nerve stumps
A combination of the previously mentioned factors.

Swelling and degradation characteristics are important inter-related physical properties of a NGC also. Materials selected for the production of NGCs should be slowly degradable into biocompatible products and have a low degree of swelling during degradation. Swelling of the NGC may occlude the lumen for regeneration or cause compression of the regenerated axons. The rate of degradation may contribute to the swelling of the NGC through the formation of breakdown products that increase the osmotic pressure within the conduit. The NGC should remain intact for the time it takes axons to regenerate across the gap and then degrade gradually with minimal swelling and foreign body reaction. This degradation rate is optimized by the copolymer ratio, in an analogous fashion to resorbable fixation plates.

Intraluminal Modifications of Single-Lumen Tubes to Enhance Regeneration

Several modifications to the single lumen hallow NGC have been investigated. These modifications are necessary when large nerve gaps exist which will exceed the inherent regenerative capacity of the peripheral nerve. When nerve gaps are short, and inherent regeneration is possible, a fibrin cable forms across the nerve gap, allowing for Schwann cell infiltration and the formation of the Bands of Bungner, which are arrays of Schwann cells and their interdigitating processes within a space circumscribed by the basement membrane (Schwann tube). Regenerating fibers then enter the gap and follow these Bands of Bungner, reach the distal end of the severed nerve, enter it, and go on to re-innervate the original target (Fig. 1). During the embryonic development of the nervous system, the developing axons are stimulated by various haptotactic (contact mediated) and chemotactic (diffusible) cues that guide growth toward their targets. Some of these signals are naturally present in a gradient concentration. Similar cues have been identified during the spontaneously occurring axon regeneration response after axonotomesis injuries. When nerve gaps are large, however, the formation of the fibrin cable and the Bands of Bungner is compromised, necessitating exogenous support to enable the regenerating fibers to cross the large nerve gap (>10 mm in rat animal models).

In attempts to maximize the regenerative capacity over larger peripheral nerve gaps, several research groups have implanted natural or synthetic materials, cells, microfibers, nanofibers, or Schwann cells seeded in matrigel to enhance the regeneration across in vitro peripheral nerve gaps. There are four essential components that are typically introduced intraluminally in NGCs to enhance NGC's outcomes.
These components are:

Growth-permissive substrates (hydrogels or nano/micro fibers)
Neurostimulatory extracellular matrix (ECM) proteins or peptides (laminin [LN-1] or LN-1 fragments)

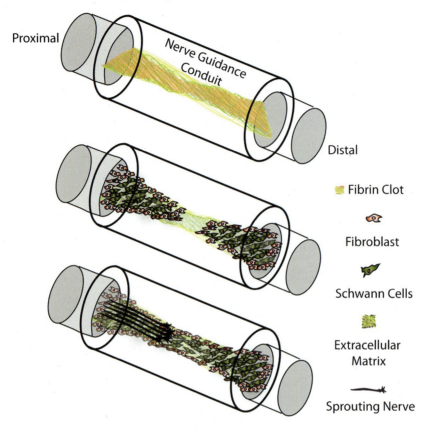

Fig. 1. Regeneration through a nerve conduit at a noncritical nerve gap.

Neurotrophic factors (bFGF, NGF, or BDNF)
Schwann cells/glial cells/stem cells.

The introduction of these factors in NGCs can provide haptotactic and chemotactic cues that enhance axonal regeneration.

Growth-permissive substrates

Growth-permissive substrates for NGCs may include intrinsic scaffolds (Fig. 2) or extracellular matrix containing gels (Fig. 3). Intrinsic scaffolds such as filaments, sponges, and multichannel nerve tubes enhance regeneration by stabilizing the fibrin matrix that is formed inside the NGC through contact guidance. The internal structure increases the intraluminal surface area and potentially concentrates growth-promoting physical and biochemical cues by facilitating endogenous Schwann cell function or facilitating local release of incorporated growth factors. However, the additional intraluminal structures may negatively influence the NGC's properties either by affecting its physical properties such as permeability or flexibility or by reducing the total open intraluminal cross-sectional area available for nerve regeneration. Therefore, the number of filaments and channels that can be put into a NGC is limited by the size (how small) at which they can be produced. Longitudinally oriented structures, such as filaments, may be used to mimic the fascicular pattern of the nerve, which consists of an intraneural plexus. This has led many researchers to pursue development of three-dimensional gels and scaffolds (collagen/laminin-containing gels).

Neurostimulatory ECM proteins or peptides

Basal lamina is a specialized extracellular matrix that acts as a scaffold for epithelial and neural cells. It contains various adhesion molecules, including laminin, fibronectin, various proteoglycans,

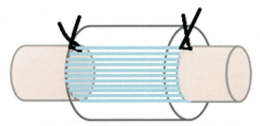

Aligned Nanofiber containing Matrices

- Poly lactide-co-glycotide (PLGA)
- Polycaprolactone (PCL)
- Collagen

Fig. 2. Schematic of aligned nanofiber containing matrices.

and collagens. Accordingly, basal lamina can be thought of as glue; on one side it is in contact with the cells, and the other side it is in contact with the surrounding connective tissue matrix, regulating the axonal growth in the distal nerve stump. ECM proteins such as collagen, laminin, and fibronectin within gels and solutions can enhance regeneration by providing haptotactic cues guiding the axon growth cones during regeneration.

The major organic component of the natural ECM of most tissues, collagen is a versatile substrate for supporting cell proliferation and regeneration. The degree to which it is cross-linked can tailor both its mechanical properties and degradation rate, and the high number of functional groups along its polypeptide backbone make it highly receptive to binding of growth factors. The use of collagen as a structural matrix for regenerating axons has been studied extensively. In 1990, Rosen revealed the true potential of collagen when he bridged a 5 mm rat peroneal nerve defect with a polyglycolic acid (PGA) conduit filled with collagen ECM. The axonal regeneration of the conduit was equal to sutured autografts at 11 to 12 months as measured by axonal counts and functional methods, although the sutured autografts demonstrated larger axonal diameters. More recent research has focused on magnetically aligning the collagen fibrils to enhance results. Dubey, in 1999, showed that there was a positive correlation between the depth and axial bias of neurite elongation and the intensity of the magnetic field used to align the collagen within conduits entubing rat dorsal root ganglia. Since this study, it has been found that magnetically aligned laminin gels perform better than collagen gels (each with embedded Schwann cells).

Laminin is another highly investigated protein of the ECM that is an abundant component of the basement membrane during the development of the embryonic nervous system. Found in the basal lamina (basement membrane) and produced by Schwann cells, it is an important adhesion molecule for growth and regeneration of neural tissue. Laminin plays a crucial role in the developing and

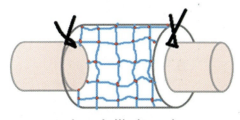

Hydrogel Filled Matrices

Natural Materials
- Agarose
- Collagen
- Chitosan
- Hyaluronic acid

Synthetic Materials
- Poly (HEMA)
- Polyethylene Glycol

Fig. 3. Schematic of natural and synthetic materials that may be used for constructing hydrogel-filled matrices.

mature central nervous system influencing cell migration, differentiation, and axonal growth. In 1985, Madison and colleagues found that introducing a gel containing 80% laminin into a nerve conduit spanning a murine-transected sciatic nerve produced, at 2 weeks, regenerating neuronal cells in the conduit compared with none in the control. In 1987, in a quantitative extension of this experiment, Madison confirmed that laminin gel significantly increased the initial rate at which axons from primary sensory and motor neurons cross a transection site. A subsequent study by the same team proved that laminin gel also could be used to extend nerve regeneration across defects thought previously too wide for this process (20–25 mm in a murine model). Since these early studies, laminin's usefulness has been demonstrated in other animal models, such as the beagle.

Fibronectin is an ECM protein that is dispersed in interstitial matrices. Although less studied, it is probably as important as laminin to support axonal outgrowth. It is composed of several rod-like domains, one of which contains a repeating sequence of peptides that regulates cell adhesion, the RGDS sequence (L-arginine, L-glycine, L-aspartic acid, and L-serine). Fibronectin has been found to play a role in axonal growth and cell migration, and the addition of fibronectin to alginate hydrogel has shown improved Schwann cell viability and growth profile in vitro. Recent studies have proposed that through the RGDS moiety, fibronectin-ligated specific integrin receptors are up-regulated in the nerve injury microenvironment. Integrins are receptors that mediate attachment between a cell and the tissues surrounding it, which may be other cells or the ECM. They also play a role in cell signaling and thereby define cellular shape, mobility, and regulate the cell cycle. Low doses of RGDS peptides were found to ligate their relevant integrin receptors to promote both axon and Schwann cell regrowth. In contrast, high doses of RGDS likely interrupt regeneration through competition for integrin receptors preventing normal interaction between axons and Schwann cells with the ECM. These findings highlight that the axon–Schwann cell interaction involves both secreted ligands and ECM molecules and signaling between the two with the nerve outgrowth zone during regeneration.

Neurotrophic factors

Certain factors are important for supporting survival, differentiation, and regeneration of nervous tissue of people and animals. Neurotrophic factors promote neuronal regrowth, sprouting, and ultimately new connections between the transected axons. This knowledge has stimulated research to evaluate their use in artificial conduits with increasing interest in the use of growth factor gradients as chemotactic cues (Fig. 4).

Growth factors are polypeptides that are produced by various cells and often show overlapping actions. Introducing growth factor therapy is a difficult task because of the high biologic activity (in pico- to nanomolar range), pleiotrophic effects (acting on various targets), and short biologic half-life (few minutes to hours) of these protein drugs. Growth factors should be therefore administered locally to achieve an adequate therapeutic effect with few adverse reactions. Localized growth factor release from NGCs can be achieved through delivery of proteins from the NGC lumen or NGC wall directly

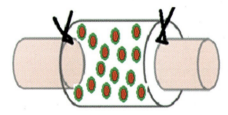

Nerve Guidance Channels with Controlled Release of Growth Factors

Growth Factors	**Carriers for Growth Factors**
•Nerve Growth Factor (NGF)	•Nanoparticles
•Neurotrophins (NT) 3,4 and 5	•Nanofibers
•Fibroblast Growth Factor (FGF)	•Microparticles
•Glial Derived Neurotrophic Factor (GDNF)	•Hydrogels
	•Lipid Microtubules

Fig. 4. Examples of growth factors and carriers for growth factors that can be placed into a nerve guidance channel.

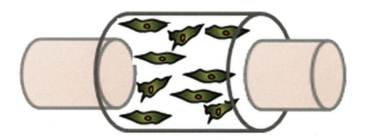

Fig. 5. Examples of support cell types, which can be used within a nerve guidance channel.

to the target nerve, seeding cells inside the NGC lumen that produce the growth factors, or using gene therapy to transfect resident cells to express a certain protein. Delivery systems are generally preferred, as the effect of growth factors is often dose-dependent and requires release over extended periods of time. Adding the factors directly to the lumen of the NGC in solution also may result in leakage from inside the tube.

NGFs are a family of neurotrophins produced by the target organs of sympathetic and sensory nerves, which play an important role in the natural process of nerve growth and regeneration. In 2003, Lee used heparin to immobilize NGF and slow its diffusion from a fibrin matrix inside a conduit

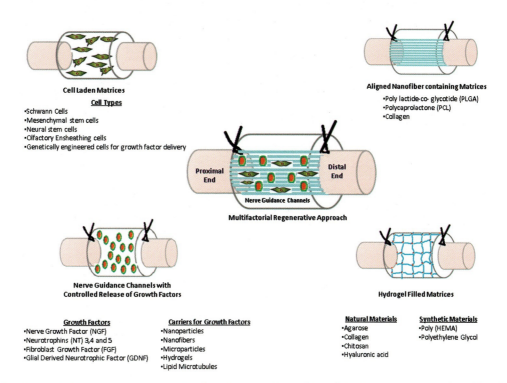

Fig. 6. A multifactor regenerative approach will combine a number of the modifications to the nerve guidance channel.

bridging a 13 mm rat sciatic nerve defect to produce similar numbers of nerve fibers compared with isograft.

Glial-derived neurotrophic factor (GDNF) promotes both sensory and motor neuron survival, and the delivery of GDNF to the peripheral nervous system has been shown to enhance regeneration following injury. Recently, Wood and colleagues found that affinity-based delivery of GDNF from a fibrin matrix in an NGC enhanced nerve regeneration in a 13 mm rat sciatic nerve defect.

Glial cells/Schwann cells/stem cells

The addition of supportive cells, especially Schwann cells, to the NGC has been extensively explored to enhance regeneration (Fig. 5). Schwann cells are glial cells of the peripheral nervous

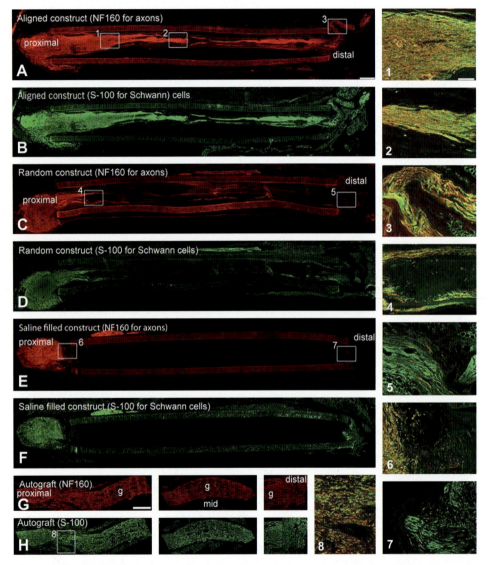

Fig. 7. Immunohistochemical analysis of nerve regeneration through implants in vivo (longitudinal section, 17 mm nerve gap). (*A, B* and *1–3*) Representative nerve regeneration through aligned fiber-based polymeric construct (aligned construct); (*C, D* and *4, 5*) nerve regeneration through random fiber-based polymeric construct (random construct). (*E, F* and *6, 7*) nerve regeneration through saline-filled polymeric construct; (*G, H* and *8*) nerve regeneration through autograft. (*A, B*) Double immunostained nerve regeneration (A, NF160) and Schwann cells infiltration from both proximal and distal nerve stump (B, S-100). Scale bar = 1 mm. Numbered images are magnified and NF160/S-100 overlapped images from boxes in (*A*). Scale bar 1/4 200 mm. (*C, D*) Double immunostained nerve regeneration (*C*) and Schwann cells (*D*). Two numbered images are from boxes in (*C*). (*E, F*) Double immunostained nerve (*E*) and Schwann cells (*F*). Numbered images are magnified and NF160/S-100 overlapped image from boxes in (*E*). (*G, H*) Double immunostained nerve regeneration (*G*) and Schwann cells (*H*). Numbered image is magnified and NF160/S-100 overlapped images from box in (*H*). Scale bar , 800 mm. *Abbreviation:* g, autograft. (*Reprinted from* Kim Y, Haftel VK, Kumar S, et al. The role of aligned polymer fiber-based constructs in the bridging of long peripheral nerve gaps. Biomaterials 2008;29:3117; with permission.)

system. They support the axons of myelinated nerves through forming the myelin sheath to provide insulation and fast conduction speed. They are also necessary for successful axonal regeneration across nerve gaps. They perform this function through production and secretion of neurotrophic factors (NGF, BDNF). Schwann cells that are devoid of contact with axons transiently proliferate, forming a cell strand called the Schwann cell column or band of Bungner within the basal lamina tube, which helps guide the regenerating axon. When regenerating axons re-enter the peripheral nerve matrix, they grow within these bands of Bungner. The Schwann cell column thus provides regenerating axons with an environment favorable for growth. If regenerating axons somehow evade the Schwann cell column and enter the connective tissue compartment, they cease to grow after elongation of only a few millimeters within the connective tissue.

Many of the neurotrophic factors that have been considered for controlled release are made by Schwann cells within this column, which serve several important roles in nerve regeneration. Thus, a logical alternative to controlled release of growth factors is to add Schwann cells directly into the lumen of the NGC. Schwann cells forming a monolayer on the inner wall of the polyethylene NGC permitted the regeneration of the axon over a 20 mm gap in the rat median nerve. Schwann cells suspended in gelatin within the lumen of polyglycolic acid conduits have supported nerve regeneration over a 40 mm gap in the tibial nerve of the rabbit. The most successful results from studies using Schwann cells have involved allogeneic or autologous Schwann cells.

Autologous Schwann cells are difficult to obtain for use as NGC luminal additives, despite recent advances, as there is only a small resource for them in the body, and the process for extracting them is relatively challenging. This difficulty could be overcome through differentiation of bone marrow stem cells into cells phenotypically similar to Schwann cells.

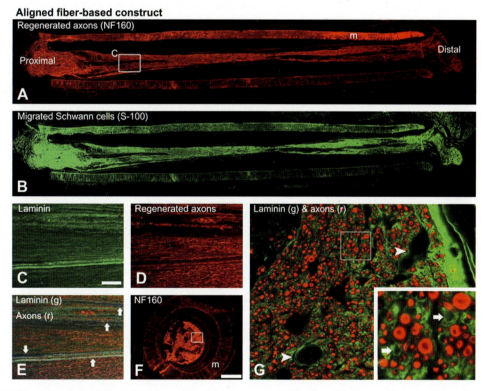

Fig. 8. Nerve regeneration through aligned construct shows presence of both migrated Schwann cells and endogenously deposited laminin protein. (A, B) Representative double immunostained nerve regeneration (A) and migrated Schwann cells from both proximal and distal nerve stump (B). (C–E) Magnified and double immunostained endogenously deposited laminin (*green, C*) and regenerating axons (*red, D*) from box in (A). (E) Triple overlapped images: laminin (*green*), axon (*red*), and aligned fiber films (*blue*). Arrows indicate fiber films. Scale bar, 200 mm. (F) Representative NF160 (a marker for axons) immunostained aligned construct (transverse cross section, 5 mm from proximal nerve stump). Scale bar, 500 mm. (G) Magnified and double immunostained regenerated axons (*red*) encircled by laminin + pocket structures (*green*) from box in (F). Arrowheads indicate blood vessels, and inset shows magnified axons and laminin + pocket structures. Arrows indicate laminin + pocket structures without regrown axon. *Abbreviation:* m, polysulfone nerve conduit. (*Reprinted from* Kim Y, Haftel VK, Kumar S, et al. The role of aligned polymer fiber-based constructs in the bridging of long peripheral nerve gaps. Biomaterials 2008;29:3117; with permission.)

Anisotropy

Anisotropy is the property of being directionally dependent, as opposed to isotropy, which implies homogeneity in all directions. Anisotropic distribution of the four components influencing peripheral nerve regeneration (growth-permissive substrate/ECM proteins/neurotrophic factors/and Schwann cells, Fig. 6) may enable faster or better regeneration, by exploiting the differential response of growth cones to changes in chemotactic features (gradients of neurotrophic factors or ECM proteins) or structural features such as oriented scaffolds versus nonoriented scaffolds (Figs. 7 and 8). When a concentration gradient of NGF is present, growth cones guide growing axons to their proper target. This suggests that gradients exploit an innate response of growth cones that is not possible with uniform, isotropic distribution of trophic factors such as NGF. Other studies have shown increased growth cone extension across gradients of laminin and NGF (Figs. 9 and 10). Likewise, oriented scaffolds using micron or nano-sized fibers within a three-dimensional gel may provide for the optimal infrastructure within the NGC.

Animal studies

As can be seen from the large number of animal studies referenced within this article, animal models are integral to designing and characterizing the ideal peripheral nerve conduit. While in most biomedical applications rats and mice are by far the two most employed laboratory animals, in nerve regeneration studies there is a clear prevalence of rat use. The anatomy of rat nerves is well established, and in general, similar to human anatomy. Rodents, however, demonstrate superior neuro-regenerative capacity compared with people and higher mammals. To recognize true differences between experimental groups, the timing of the outcome measurement is crucial. Clinical correlation can only be made with earlier time points. Late time points may show experimental groups to be equivalent due to the blow-through effect, in which the superlative rodent regenerative capacity masks the true differences between the groups.

In rat models, it is imperative that two factors are involved, namely a gap greater than 10 mm (critical defect) if the sciatic nerve is used, and controls involving autografts. If regeneration in such models is successful, it is crucial to test the engineered scaffold in a larger animal (such as the rabbit)

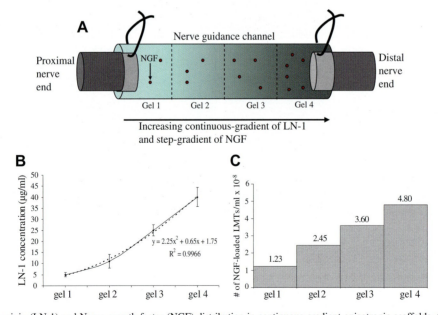

Fig. 9. Laminin (LN-1) and Nerve growth factor (NGF) distribution in continuous-gradient anisotropic scaffolds. (*A*) is an A nerve guidance channel (NGC) connected to nerve ends, with four layers of gels in it. LN-1 gradient is smooth (*B*), as determined by LN-1 enzyme-linked immunoassay (ELISA), while NGF-loaded lipid microtubules (LMTs) are distributed in a step-gradient fashion (*C*). With time, NGF will diffuse out of the LMTs and form a smooth gradient. (*Reprinted from* MC Dodla, R.V. Bellamkonda. Biomaterials 2008;29:33–46; with permission.)

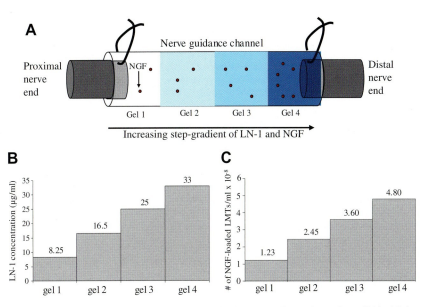

Fig. 10. Laminin (LN-1) and nerve growth factor (NGF) distribution in step-gradient anisotropic scaffolds. (*A*) is a schematic of a NGC connected to nerve ends, with four layers of gels. The darker shades of gel represent increasing concentration of LN-1. (*B*) Gel 4 has higher concentration of LN-1. (*C*) Gel 4 also has a higher number of NGF-loaded lipid microtubules (LMTs).

with gaps greater than 40 mm to further validate the regenerative strategy. The possibility that sensory nerves can have different regeneration patterns should be also be taken into consideration in clinical translation of the experimental results gained from in vivo models using somatic mixed nerve models, as this is especially applicable to peripheral sensory branches of the trigeminal nerve such as the lingual and inferior alveolar.

The method of analyses to determine success is also important. Most investigations of peripheral nerve regeneration employ anatomic and histologic criteria, yet it is more ideal to include a functional evaluation of the quality of the regenerated nerve distal to the gap site. This can be accomplished through measurement of the number and quality of the neuromuscular junctions, electrophysiology, or also with simultaneous and sequential retrograde tracing. In the most commonly used model, the rat sciatic nerve, two different tracers can be applied simultaneously to the tibial and peroneal nerve branches to determine the dispersion of regenerating axons originating from the same neuron, or the two tracers can be applied to the same nerve branch before and after repair to determine the correct direction of regenerating axons.

Summary/Future strategies

Although resorbable NGCs have been developed for peripheral nerve grafting, there has been little published on their use as a material for trigeminal nerve repair. Advances in engineered guidance channels and modifications to the single-lumen conduit with growth-permissive substrates, ECM proteins, neurotrophic factors, and supportive Schwann or stem cells, and anisotropic placement of these within the NGC may translate from animal models to clinical human use in the future. A great deal of research is still needed to optimize the presently available NGCs, and their use in peripheral trigeminal nerve repair and regeneration remains yet to be explored. Bioengineered NGCs and additives remain promising alternatives to autogenous nerve grafting in the future. They can incorporate all of the developing strategies for peripheral nerve regeneration that develop in concert with the ever-increasing understanding of regenerative mechanisms. The use of nanomaterials also may resolve the numerous problems associated with traditional conduit limitations by better mimicking the properties of natural tissues. Since cells directly interact with nanostructured ECM proteins, the biomimetic features of anisotropic-designed nanomaterials coupled with luminal additive ECMs, neurotrophic factors, and Schwann cells may provide for great progress in peripheral nerve regeneration.

Further readings

Archibald SJ, Krarup C, Shefner J, et al. A collagen-based nerve guide conduit for peripheral nerve repair: an electrophysiological study of nerve regeneration in rodents and nonhuman primates. J Comp Neurol 1991;306(4):685.

Bellamkonda RV. Peripheral nerve regeneration: an opinion on channels, scaffolds and anisotropy. Biomaterials 2006;27:3515.

Brenner MJ, Moradzadeh A, Myckatyn TM, et al. Role of timing in assessment of nerve regeneration. Microsurgery 2008; 28:265.

Bunge RP. Expanding roles for the Schwann cell: ensheathment, myelination, trophism, and regeneration. Curr Opin Neurobiol 1993;3:805.

Chaudry V, Glass JD, Griffin JW. Wallerian degeneration in peripheral nerve disease. Neurol Clin 1992;10:613.

Chiono V, Tonda-Turo C, Ciardelli G. Artificial scaffolds for peripheral nerve reconstruction. Essays on peripheral nerve repair and regeneration (Elsevier). Int Rev Neurobiol 2009;87:173.

DeRuiter GC, Malessy M, Yaszemski MJ, et al. Designing ideal conduits for nerve repair. Neurosurg Focus 2009;26(2):E5.

Dodla MC, Bellamkonda RV. Differences between the effect of anisotropic and isotropic laminin and nerve growth factor presenting scaffolds on nerve regeneration across long peripheral nerve gaps. Biomaterials 2008;29:33.

Dodla MC, Bellamkonda RV. Anisotropic scaffolds facilitate enhanced neurite extension in vitro. J Biomed Mater Res 2006; 78:213.

Evans GR. Peripheral nerve injury: a review and approach to tissue engineered constructs. Anat Rec 2001;263:396.

Giannini C, Dyck PJ. The fate of Schwann cell basement membranes in permanently transected nerves. J Neuropathol Exp Neurol 1990;49:550.

Hudson TW, Evans GR, Schmidt CE. Engineering strategies for peripheral nerve repair. Clin Plast Surg 1999;26:617.

Ide C. Peripheral nerve regeneration. Neurosci Res 1996;25:101.

Kim Y, Haftel VK, Kumar S, et al. The role of aligned polymer fiber-based constructs in the bridging of long peripheral nerve gaps. Biomaterials 2008;29:3117.

Lee AC, Yu VM, Lowe JB, et al. Controlled release of nerve growth factor enhances sciatic nerve regeneration. Exp Neurol 2003;184:295.

Madison RD, da Silva CF, Dikkes P, et al. Increased rate of peripheral nerve regeneration using bioabsorbable nerve guides and a laminin-containing gel. Exp Neurol 1985;88:767.

Madison RD, da Silva CF, Dikkes P. Entubulation repair with protein additives increases the maximum nerve gap distance successfully bridged with tubular prostheses. Brain Res 1988;447:325.

Moore AM, Kasukurthi R, Magill CK, et al. Limitations of conduits in peripheral nerve repair. Hand 2009;4:180.

Moradzadeh A, Borschel GH, Luciano JP, et al. The impact of motor and sensory nerve architecture on nerve regeneration. Exp Neurol 2008;21:370.

Nichols CM, Brenner MJ, Fox IK, et al. Effects of motor versus sensory nerve grafts on peripheral nerve regeneration. Exp Neurol 2004;190:347.

Pfister LA, Papaloizos M, Merkle HP, et al. Nerve conduits and growth factor delivery in peripheral nerve repair. J Peripher Nerv Syst 2007;12:65.

Pitta MC, Wolford LM, Mehra P, et al. Use of Gore-Tex tubing as a conduit for inferior alveolar and lingual nerve repair: Experience with 6 cases. J Oral Maxillofac Surg 2001;59:493.

Pogrel MA, McDonald AR, Kaban LB. Gore-Tex tubing as a conduit for repair of lingual and inferior alveolar nerve continuity defects: a preliminary report. J Oral Maxillofac Surg 1998;56:319.

Politis MJ, Ederle K, Spencer PS. Tropism in nerve regeneration in vivo. Attraction of regenerating axons by diffusible factors derived from cells in distal nerve stumps of transected peripheral nerves. Brain Res 1982;253:1.

Richardson PM. Neurotrophic factors in regeneration. Curr Opin Neurobiol 1991;1:401.

Rosen JM, Padilla JA, Nguyen KD, et al. Artificial nerve graft using collagen as an extracellular matrix for repair compared with sutured autograft in the rat model. Ann Plast Surg 1990;25:375.

Rosen JM, Padilla JA, Nguyen KD, et al. Artificial nerve graft using glycolide trimethylene carbonate as a nerve conduit filled with collagen compared to sutured autograft in a rat model. J Rehabil Res Dev 1992;29:1.

Rosen JM, Pham HN, Abraham G, et al. Artificial nerve graft compared to autograft in a rat model. J Rehabil Res Dev 1989;26:1.

Wolford L. Considerations in nerve repair. Proc (Bayl Univ Med Cent) 2003;16:152.

Wood MD, Moore AM, Hunter DA, et al. Affinity based release of glial-derived neurotrophic factor from fibrin matrices enhances sciatic nerve regeneration. Acta Biomater 2009;5:959.

Zuo J, Hernandez YJ, Muir D. Chondroitin Sulfate proteoglycan with neurite- inhibiting activity is up regulated following peripheral nerve injury. J Neurobiol 1998;34:41.

Moving?

Make sure your subscription moves with you!

To notify us of your new address, find your **Clinics Account Number** (located on your mailing label above your name), and contact customer service at:

Email: journalscustomerservice-usa@elsevier.com

800-654-2452 (subscribers in the U.S. & Canada)
314-447-8871 (subscribers outside of the U.S. & Canada)

Fax number: 314-447-8029

**Elsevier Health Sciences Division
Subscription Customer Service
3251 Riverport Lane
Maryland Heights, MO 63043**

*To ensure uninterrupted delivery of your subscription, please notify us at least 4 weeks in advance of move.